COMMON DISORDERS OF THE
TEMPOROMANDIBULAR JOINT

A DENTAL PRACTITIONER HANDBOOK
SERIES EDITED BY DONALD D. DERRICK, DDS LDS RCS

COMMON DISORDERS OF THE TEMPOROMANDIBULAR JOINT

HUGH D. OGUS
BDS (Lond), FDS RCS (Eng)
Consultant Oral Surgeon, Basingstoke District Hospital

and

The late PAUL A. TOLLER
FDS RCS (Eng)
*Late Consultant Oral Surgeon, Mount Vernon Hospital,
Northwood and Canadian Red Cross Hospital, Taplow*

With a Chapter by
JAMES V. MANZIONE
MD DMD
*Assistant Professor, Department of Radiology, University of Rochester,
School of Medicine and Dentistry, Rochester, New York*

With a Foreword by
DANIEL M. LASKIN
DDS MS
*Professor and Head of Department of Oral and
Maxillofacial Surgery, University of Illinois, Chicago*

Second edition

WRIGHT

BRISTOL
1986

Published by

John Wright & Sons Ltd, Techno House, Redcliffe Way, Bristol, BS1 6NX, England

First edition, 1981
Second edition, 1986

British Library Cataloguing in Publication Data

Ogus, Hugh D.
    Common disorders of the temporomandibular joint. —
    2nd ed. — (A Dental practitioner handbook; v.26)
    1. Temporomandibular joint — Diseases
    I. Title   II. Toller, Paul A.   III. Manzione,
    James V.   IV. Series
    617'.522   RK470

ISBN 0 7236 0874 1

Printed in Great Britain by
Henry Ling Ltd, Dorset Press, Dorchester

To
MAGGIE

PREFACE TO THE SECOND EDITION

Since the publication of the first edition of this book there have been several important advances in our understanding of temporomandibular joint disorders. These concern the anatomy and pathophysiology of the joint and are due to the new imaging techniques that have become more readily available to both clinician and researcher.

To take account of the advances, Chapter 3 in the original text, The Examination, has been split into two chapters. The first deals with the clinical examination and the second with radiographic evaluation. The latter has been written by James Manzione who, for several years, has specialized in arthrography, tomography and other imaging techniques for the temporomandibular joint.

In Chapter 5, I have added a section on electromyography prepared by Richard Juniper, Oral and Maxillofacial Surgeon from Oxford.

The evidence contained in these changes and additions has altered my appreciation of the pathophysiology of the joint, especially with regard to meniscal displacement. However, it supports and even enhances the fundamental concept upon which this book is based, that most common disorders of the temporomandibular joint are due to stress-induced neuromuscular overload.

H.D.O.

PREFACE TO THE FIRST EDITION

Paul Toller died on the 13th July 1977 after a long and painful illness. His death at an early age was a tragic loss, not only for his family and friends, but also to the clinical and scientific communities of medicine and dentistry. His ever-active and enquiring mind was continually involved with a multiplicity of interests, both clinical and non-clinical but perhaps he became best known for his research into the conditions and diseases of the temporomandibular joint.

About a year before his death he had been asked by John Wright & Sons Ltd if he would consider writing a book for their successful Dental Practitioner Handbook series. He readily agreed and although never fully deciding on a title began to compose his ideas and indeed produce outline texts for several chapters and sections.

On account of my close association with Paul Toller in the latter years of his life, and also of my interest and similar ideas concerning the problems of the temporomandibular joint, I was approached by Donald Derrick, the editor of the series, with a request to carry on the project.

I decided to limit the scope of the book and deal only with the common conditions that affect the joint. The concepts that I have described show the obvious influence that Paul Toller has had on my understanding of the temporomandibular joint, but in some instances I have extended his ideas, principally along the lines on which he himself was working. I must surely also acknowledge the abundance of literature, references, diagrams and photographic illustrations that he had accumulated over the years, and which were made available to me by his wife Dorothy and his colleagues at Mount Vernon Hospital. Without this assistance my task would have been much greater.

H. D. O.

ACKNOWLEDGEMENTS

Many people have assisted me in producing this book and in particular I would like to express my gratitude to Dorothy Kramer and Gordon Fordyce for allowing me access to much of Paul Toller's material; Robert Toy and Ronald Blake from the Photography Departments at Basingstoke and Mount Vernon Hospitals; my son, Michael, for his drawings and diagrams; Peter Banks for the photographs of the closed condylotomy procedure and the Editors of the *British Dental Journal,* the *Journal of the Royal Society of Medicine* and the *British Journal of Oral Surgery* for permission to publish many of the illustrations. My thanks also to Neville Barker for his assistance in writing the section on Hypnotherapy. Finally, I would like to thank Brian O'Riorden for his valuable criticism of the text and Jill Franklin, my secretary, for typing and retyping the manuscript.

CONTENTS

FOREWORD

Daniel M. Laskin DDS MS

Although the pathological conditions that affect the temporomandibular joint are the same as those which affect other joints of the body, the unusual anatomical and functional characteristics of this structure often lead to unique clinical manifestations and growth disturbances that are not seen when these conditions occur in other areas. Added to this already complex situation is the frequent occurrence of secondary pathological alterations in the temporomandibular joint resulting from psychophysiologically generated changes in the associated masticatory muscles. Thus the dental practitioner is faced with a variety of conditions of diverse aetiology, often producing quite similar signs and symptoms, that are not only difficult to diagnose but also difficult to treat.

Much of the current controversy regarding the management of temporomandibular joint disorders is related to the development of concepts of aetiology based on the effects of empirical therapy rather than derived from sound biological principles. The situation is further compounded by the failure of many clinicians to recognize and distinguish between the organic disorders and those of psychophysiological origin, and to understand the relationship between them. The end result is often the propagation of empiricism and the inappropriate care of patients.

The authors of this text have avoided these pitfalls by clearly defining the diagnostic criteria for the conditions discussed and basing their proposed therapy on a careful consideration of biological concepts, research data and logical reasoning, rather than on historical information and personal opinion. As a consequence, a treatment philosophy is developed that emphasizes conservatism, and reserves surgery only as a last resort. Although not every practitioner may agree with, or wish to adopt, all of the proposed forms of treatment, the basic discussion of joint anatomy and physiology provided by the authors should at least enable them to evaluate their own therapeutic procedures and to eliminate those without a rational basis.

Despite its brevity, this book contains a wealth of valuable basic and clinical information about the temporomandibular joint that has not been previously published. It is unfortunate that the untimely death of Paul Toller brought to an end a brilliant career in research that could have added much more to our understanding of this complex region. Hugh Ogus is to be commended for his continuation of this work and his own personal contributions to it. It was my privilege to have known Paul Toller as a colleague and a friend. He has left his mark on our profession in many ways, and his passing has not gone unnoticed.

INTRODUCTION

The triad of symptoms—clicking, locking and pain—comprise by far the most common complaint associated with the temporomandibular joint. The world literature contains a prodigious number of references to this well-recognized problem which has been described under a variety of headings. Probably the most widely accepted are the terms 'pain-dysfunction syndrome' (Schwartz, 1956) and 'myofascial pain-dysfunction' (Laskin, 1969).

More numerous than the titles, however, are the hypotheses relating to the aetiology of the symptoms and the variety of techniques that are employed in their management. A report (Ogus, 1979) described the case of a 20-year-old female with a two-year history of a bilateral temporomandibular joint disorder. Over that period, she had received the following treatment: (1) Bite appliances (three types); (2) Short-wave diathermy; (3) Remedial exercises; (4) Ultrasonic therapy; (5) Indomethacin (Indocid, Indocin—anti-arthritic); (6) Diazepam (Valium —sedative and muscle relaxant); (7) Removal of impacted third molars; and (8) Intracapsular corticosteroids. The problem was finally treated surgically, with a high condylar arthroplasty to one joint and a condylotomy to the other.

The diversity of these widely practised techniques, however, poses a number of questions; how and why do they all work, and when should one method be employed in preference to another? Is it possible that we are dealing with several separate disorders; or are the symptoms merely different manifestations of the same underlying condition?

It would seem that the management of the problem is largely empirical and, in common with any other medical condition, a reasoned approach cannot be devised until its aetiology and natural history are fully understood. There are several contemporary philosophies and the authors are well aware of the theories that they expound. The role of the occlusion in the aetiology of the disorder and meniscal displacement are both examples of the many contentious issues that surround the subject. Thus the account that is given in the following chapters contains ideas that are acceptable to some experts in the field yet are abhored by others.

Finally, the approach may be criticized on account of its psycho-logical emphasis, but then psychology plays such a large part in everyday clinical medical and dental practice. Some of the concepts remain hypothetical but it is an attempt to provide a rational explanation as well as a clinical guide to the common disorders of the temporo-mandibular joint.

CHAPTER 1

THE TEMPOROMANDIBULAR JOINT

Many of the concepts discussed in this book have been evolved only over the last decade as a consequence of an increase in our knowledge of the anatomy and physiology of the joint. Furthermore an appreciation of the development, structure and function of the mandibular joint is fundamental to the understanding and management of the conditions with which it is afflicted. Not only have colleagues in the clinical disciplines of medicine and dentistry been involved in the research and debate on these topics, but so also have workers in other fields, such as physical and biological chemistry, and even the mechanical sciences of tribology* and engineering.

DEVELOPMENT
Embryological Development
In evolutionary terms the temporomandibular joint is a secondary development. The primary or reptilian type (*Fig.* 1.1*a*), which is formed at the dorsal end of Meckel's cartilage, is represented in man as the joint between the malleus and incus of the middle ear and hence reflects the adaptation of the bones of the primitive jaw to sound conduction. This rather complicated evolution is responsible for the late embryonic appearance of the mandibular, compared with other synovial joints.

Most synovial joints have appeared by the 7th week *in utero* as a cavitation within the single blastema from which both adjoining endochondrial bones develop. The temporomandibular joint, on the other hand, arises from two widely separated centres that grow towards one another (*Fig.* 1.1*b*). By the 12th week *in utero* the developing squamous portion of the temporal bone and the secondary condylar cartilage which forms on the dorsal aspect of the developing mandibular ramus are in close apposition. A pair of clefts develop in the interposed condensation of the mesenchyme, forming upper and lower joint cavities and thus defining the meniscus (*Fig.* 1.1*c*).

The tissues comprising the meniscus at this stage are in continuity anteriorly with the developing lateral pterygoid muscle and posteriorly with the perichondrium covering the part of Meckel's cartilage which is differentiating into the malleus. The anterior extension remains, but the posterior only persists until fusion of the petrous and tympanic ring

---

*Tribology — study of friction, wear and lubrication.

1

portions of the temporal bone, thus closing the joint off from the middle ear.

From about the 12th week *in utero* there is a rapid growth of the condylar cartilage which forms a cone-shaped mass, tapering anteriorly as far as the crypt of the second deciduous molar. Gradually the cartilage is replaced by membranous bone, although its posterior part persists in the condyle as the site of active growth until the end of the second decade. Its continued presence, therefore, provides the means of further adaptation of condylar morphology in response to functional and environmental changes.

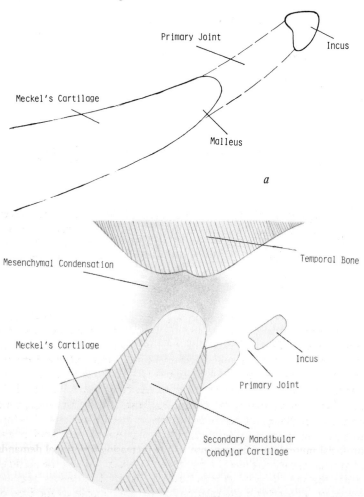

Fig. 1.1. (*see opposite*)

2

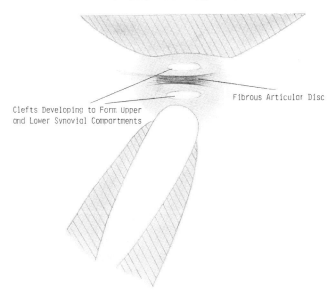

Fibrous Articular Disc

Clefts Developing to Form Upper
and Lower Synovial Compartments

Fig. 1.1. Diagrammatic representation of temporomandibular joint development (modified after Sperber). *a,* The primary joint; *b,* The bony elements; *c,* The capsule and meniscus.

The capsule develops by condensation of the surrounding mesenchyme which progressively isolates the joint with its synovial membrane from the surrounding tissues. At birth it is the sole means of stability of the joint, the glenoid fossa being almost flat and the articular eminence having not yet developed.

Postnatal Development

Postnatally the condyle continues to grow by endochondral ossification but its exact role in the further growth of the mandible has been subject to controversy. Traditionally the condylar cartilage was thought to provide the forward and downward displacement of the mandible during its development, behaving in a somewhat similar manner to the epiphyseal plate of a long bone. However, since the evolution of the functional matrix theory (Moss and Rankow, 1968), this concept has now been challenged. This theory proposed that the mandible develops to a size determined not only genetically but also by the stimuli of the orofacial musculature in response to the increasing functional demands of growth. It follows therefore that the subarticular zone of the cartilage is not the site of active growth but rather that of secondary adaptive responses, maintaining the relationship of the condyle to the base of the skull as it expands laterally, and of remodelling changes whereby

3

the shape of the condyle is altered in response to gradual changes in its functional environment.

Blackwood (1976) considers the problem in a different manner, suggesting that within the controversy the two elements of mandibular development are being confused, namely the contribution by the cartilage to growth in height of the mandibular ramus and growth of the main body of the mandible which is entirely in membrane bone. The facial deformity resulting from unilateral hyperplasia of the condyle is evidence of considerable growth potential in the condylar cartilage, but where agenesis of the condyle occurs, the body of the mandible is still found to develop to a considerable extent. Even so, there seems to be no doubt as to the inherent adaptive potential of the condyle which remains throughout life.

As previously stated, the upper bony element of the joint, the temporal component, is quite flat at birth. Gradually, mainly by apposition of the bone in the region of the articular eminence, but also by some resorption in the fossa, the adult contour is formed. At the same time, in response to function, the characteristic form and flexibility of the meniscus are established by re-orientation of the constituent fibres.

STRUCTURE OF THE TEMPOROMANDIBULAR JOINT

The temporomandibular joint has many structural features that make it a unique diarthrosis. These must be considered at all times in relation to its complex functional activities for which it is ideally adapted.

Articulating Surfaces

The bony element of the joint is made up of the mandibular condyle below and the articular surface of the temporal bone above. The adult condyle is roughly elliptical in shape, the long axis (mediolateral) being angled backwards at between 15° and 33° to the frontal plane (*Fig. 1.2*) (Berry, 1960). The mediolateral dimension varies between 13 and 25 mm and the anteroposterior width between 5·5 and 16 mm (Oberg et al., 1971). The articular surface of the temporal bone is made up of the glenoid fossa, as far posteriorly as the squamotympanic fissure, and the convexity of the articular eminence anteriorly. Its medial margin is the suture between the squamous portion of the temporal bone and the greater wing of the sphenoid.

Unlike other arthroses, whose articulating surfaces are covered with hyaline cartilage, those of the temporomandibular (and clavicular end of the sternoclavicular) joints are lined with fibrous tissue. This difference has been attributed to the membranous ossification in which the mandible, temporal bone and clavicle are formed, compared with the endochondrial ossification of the long bones.

4

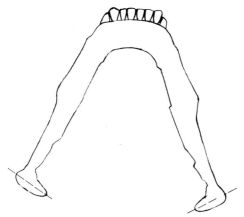

Fig. 1.2. The angulation of the mediolateral axis of the condyle to the frontal plane.

The fibrous layer covering the posterior aspect of the adult condyle is very thin and applied directly to the underlying bone, but over the convexity it becomes thicker with an intervening layer of fibrocartilage (*Fig.* 1.3*b*). In section, the fibrous tissue can be resolved into an outer layer in which the collagen bundles run parallel to the articulating surface, and an inner layer in which they run obliquely. Situated amongst the fibrous tissue and generally following the same directions are abundant elastic fibres. Their function is not yet clear although Miles and Dawson (1962) have suggested the following. The mucopolysaccharide content of the fibrous tissue layer of the mandibular joint is far lower than that of the equivalent hyaline cartilage layer of other synovial arthroses. Since the presence of these substances, and chondroitin sulphate in particular, is partially responsible for the resilience of the hyaline cartilage, it may be that the elastic fibres confer the same property on the articular fibrous tissue.

Beneath the condylar articular surface lies a thin band of cells, the intermediate or proliferative zone (*Fig.* 1.3*a*). In older joints this layer may not be very distinct but the cells of this zone are capable of proliferative activity throughout life and, as will be discussed later, play an important part in the remodelling and repair of the articular surface. The underlying hypertrophic or fibrocartilage zone may show some mineralization close to the bone, but the amount is variable.

In the growing condyle the proliferative zone is very active and thus much wider. The changes in the hypertrophic zone are similar to those accompanying ossification in cartilage elsewhere in the body; these are matrix production, cell hypertrophy and mineralization.

5

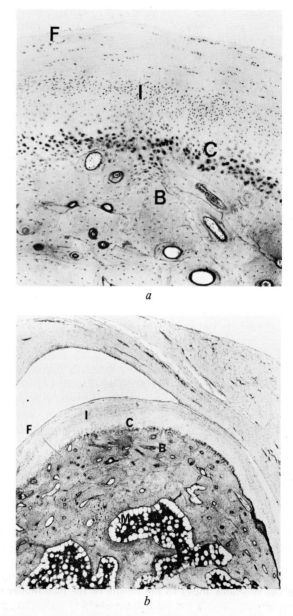

Fig. 1.3. Histological section through the adult condyle. F, Fibrous outer zone; I, Intermediate proliferative zone; C, Fibrocartilaginous zone; B, Bone. *a,* × 57. *b,* × 16.

The bony cavity of the glenoid fossa is quite thin and lined only with a narrow layer of fibrous tissue. Anteriorly, however, over the articular eminence and complimentary to the convexity of the condyle, the fibrous layer becomes wider. Interposed here, between it and the bone, is again a layer of fibrocartilage with a similar histological structure to that of the condylar surface.

Joint Capsule

The joint is enclosed within a funnel-shaped capsule which, although somewhat deficient anteriorly is circumferentially attached to the rim of the glenoid fossa and the articular eminence of the temporal bone above and to the neck of the condyle below. The entire lateral aspect of the condyle is thickened to form the main stabilizing ligament of the joint (the temporomandibular ligament) but this should be regarded as part of the capsule and inseparable from it (*Fig.* 1.4).

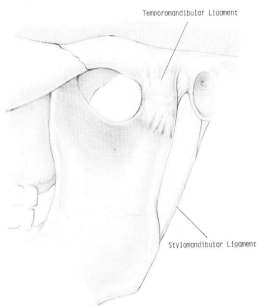

Temporomandibular Ligament

Stylomandibular Ligament

Fig. 1.4. The capsule of the temporomandibular joint from the lateral aspect.

Medially the weak sphenomandibular ligament passes from the spine of the sphenoid above to the lingula of the mandibular foramen below but is quite separate from the capsule (*Fig.* 1.5). Posteriorly the stylomandibular ligament is no more than a band of thickened cervical fascia which stretches from the apex of the styloid process to the posterior edge of the mandibular ramus.

7

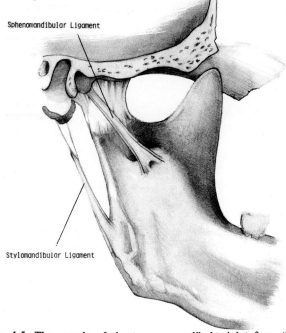

Sphenomandibular Ligament

Stylomandibular Ligament

Fig. 1.5. The capsule of the temporomandibular joint from the medial aspect.

Meniscus

The meniscus (disc) divides the joint capsule into upper and lower compartments or cavities. Although chondroid cells have been identified in its structure (Matthews and Moffett, 1974), the meniscus itself is formed of avascular collagen. This imparts a flexibility, enabling it to stabilize the condyle against the temporal articulation, even though its shape must vary as it translates forward from the glenoid fossa to the convexity of the eminence. A stiff cartilaginous structure could not serve this function. The disc is not of uniform thickness (Rees, 1954). There is a thin central zone with thicker anterior and posterior bands (Rees, 1954).

The meniscus is attached tightly to the periosteum at the medial and lateral poles of the condyle (*Fig.* 1.6*a*). Anteriorly the capsule, meniscus and condyle blend with the tendons of the lateral pterygoid muscle (*Fig.* 1.6*b*). The superior head of the lateral pterygoid, all except for a few strands, is attached to the meniscus while the larger inferior head is inserted into the neck of the condyle. Between these insertions and just anterior to the capsule lies the lateral pterygoid

8

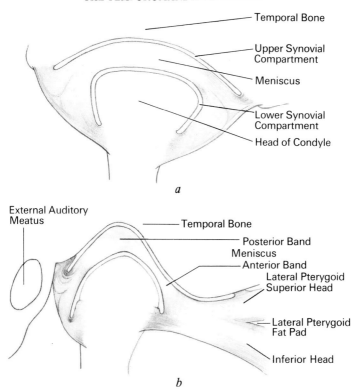

Fig. 1.6. Sections through the temporomandibular joint. *a,* Anterior view; *b,* Lateral view.

fat pad. These attachments are such that they allow the rotation component of mandibular opening that occurs in the lower joint cavity. The sliding component, the movement that takes place mainly in the upper joint compartment, is limited by the posterior attachment of the meniscus. This is a bilaminar structure. The superior lamella is attached to the posterior margin of the glenoid fossa at the squamotympanic fissure and is composed of fibroelastic tissue. The inferior lamella, which is non-elastic, blends with the periosteum at the back of the condyle. The area between the lamellae is filled with loose fibrofatty tissue richly penetrated by a venous plexus, so as to provide a soft flexible tissue which may be drawn into the regions vacated by the condyle during its functional excursions.

The shape and relationship of the meniscus to the articulating bony surfaces is illustrated in *Fig.* 1.7.

9

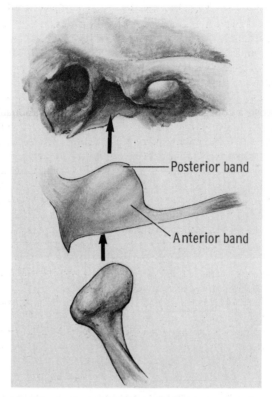

Fig. 1.7. The head of the condyle is enveloped by the meniscus, with the superior head of the lateral pterygoid inserted into its anterior edge. The meniscus may represent the modified tendon of insertion of the muscle. (Reproduced by permission of the *Br. J. Oral Maxillofac. Surg.*)

Synovial Membrane

At birth, synovial membrane covers all the internal surfaces of the joint including the meniscus. As function commences, this lining is lost from all the articulating surfaces, remaining only on the inner aspects of the capsule. Thus the synovia are continuous with the fibrous tissue covering the disc and the surface of the condyle and temporal articulation, although there is a transitional zone with intermediate grades of structure between those of the typical membrane and the articular surface.

Some areas of the synovia, especially where they line loose connective tissue in the anterior and posterior limits of both cavities (the capsular sulci), are thrown up into finger-like projections, the synovial villi.

10

These increase the flexibility of the inner surfaces of the capsule enabling the changes in the shape of the disc and sulci to occur during normal movements. Since they also increase the surface area of the synovial membrane, the villi may have the effect of promoting the distribution of synovial fluid over the articulating surfaces.

Synovial membrane consists of two cell layers, the intima and the subintima. The latter is basically formed of loose vascular connective tissue although a collagen and elastic component is occasionally found. This is said to prevent the formation of excessively redundant folds of membrane which might otherwise become entrapped between the articular surfaces. The intimal layer, directly adjacent to the joint cavity contains two principal cell types (Hamerman et al., 1970). 'Type A' cells, characterized by a surface layer of fine filaments and a pronounced Golgi apparatus (typical of a macrophage) are more abundant than 'type B' cells which have fewer vacuoles, a smaller Golgi apparatus and a high proportion of rough endoplasmic reticulum. The exact function of each cell type is not yet clear but the functions of the synovia as a whole are thought to be:

a. Regulatory — controlling the entry of nutrients, electrolytes and other materials into the synovial fluid;

b. Secretory — the intimal cells secrete a proportion of the synovial fluid components; and

c. Phagocytic — it is thought that the 'type A' cells help debride the joint cavity.

Nerve Supply

The innervation of the temporomandibular joint consists of a dense plexus of unmyelinated fibres that weaves throughout the fibrous capsule and related fibrofatty tissue (Wyke, 1976). The plexus is most dense in the posterior portion of the structure. The small-diameter afferent pain fibres enter the regionally related articular branches of the auriculotemporal, masseteric, deep temporal and sometimes lateral pterygoid nerves, whence they pass into the sensory root and spinal tract of the trigeminal nerve.

It must be stressed that as in all other synovial joints there are no nerve endings of any type in the fibrous articular surface, the fibrocartilage, disc or synovia. These structures therefore are certainly not the cause of primary articular pain, which is probably only produced by mechanical or chemical irritation of the sensitive capsular tissues surrounding the joint.

Nutrition

The blood supply to the joint is through the internal maxillary artery, principally via its deep auricular branch. Much of the structure, however (the meniscus, the fibrous and fibrocartilage layers) is mainly avascular and depends for its metabolism on diffusion from the deeper bone and superficially, the synovial fluid.

Some Anatomical Relations

The temporomandibular joint is surrounded on all sides by important anatomical structures which may be relevant both from diagnostic and surgical aspects. Examples of the former are numerous as any clinician dealing with the problem of diagnosing facial pain is only too well aware. From the point of view of the surgeon, however, the relationship of many of the structures varies in respect to the joint, thus invalidating a rigid description of its surgical anatomy.

Deep to the joint lies the first part of the internal maxillary artery, which passes forward horizontally between the neck of the condyle and the sphenomandibular ligament, giving off several branches including the inferior alveolar (dental) artery.

Above the joint, the roof of the glenoid fossa is thin and corresponds medially to the most lateral part of the floor of the middle cranial fossa, and laterally to the roof of the zygomatic process of the temporal bone. The mandibular joint is thus closely related to the meninges and cranial contents.

Posteriorly lies the cartilaginous part of the external auditory meatus which may be partially separated from the joint by a medial extension of the parotid gland.

Posterolaterally to the joint lies the superficial temporal artery and veins, and the auriculotemporal nerve which winds around behind the neck of the condyle. More superficially and covering most of its outer aspect, is the upper pole of the parotid gland, enclosed within its capsule of deep cervical fascia. The most important structure in this area is the facial nerve which enters the posteromedial surface of the gland, level with the lower edge of the tragus (*Fig.* 1.8). Within the gland it splits up to provide motor nerves to the facial muscles. Its temporal and zygomatic branches are somewhat variable in their courses but generally one or more of their strands cross upwards and forwards, across the lateral aspect of the joint capsule but within the parotid fascia. The surgical significance of the anatomy of the facial nerve will be discussed further in Chapter 7.

Ultramicroscopy

Ultramicroscopic examination of the articular tissue of the condyle reveals a dense interlacing meshwork of collagen fibril bundles interposed with fibrocytes (*Fig.* 1.9*b*). The density of the collagen here is greater than in the hyaline cartilage of other joint surfaces. The orientation of the bundles is not haphazard, the decussations being arranged in such a way that the majority are tangential to the surface.

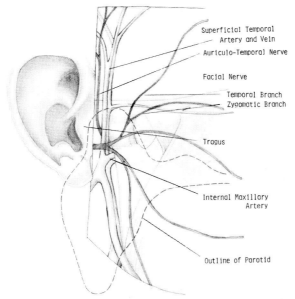

Superficial Temporal Artery and Vein

Auriculo-Temporal Nerve

Facial Nerve

Temporal Branch
Zygomatic Branch

Tragus

Internal Maxillary Artery

Outline of Parotid

Fig. 1.8. The relationship of the temporomandibular joint to the parotid gland, facial nerve and other anatomical structures.

The collagen fibrils are not of uniform diameter but seem to be composed of two groups—small diameter fibrils, about 30–50 nm in thickness, interspaced with large diameter fibrils of 150–200 nm. The proportion of small to large fibrils is variable. Occasionally, among the collagen, are found straight elastic fibres.

The fibroblasts are long spindle-shaped cells (not flattened as suggested by light microscopy) with many blade-like processes of plasma membrane which intrude between adjacent fasciculi of the collagen bundles and for whose formation they are presumably responsible. Generally the fibre bundles run parallel to the long axes of the cells. In the transverse section the fibroblasts appear irregularly star-shaped due to section of their processes. Near the articular surface, the cells have a smaller proportion of cytoplasm and contain fewer organelles then in the deeper layers. Throughout, however, the nuclei are of the same size and shape and retain their integrity even close to the surface.

Occupying the space between the individual collagen fibrils, bundles and cells, is the ground substance or intercellular matrix. It is only a very small percentage of the total bulk of the structure and cannot be visualized in an electron micrograph on account of its low electron density. It is known to be composed of a complex sulphur-containing

13

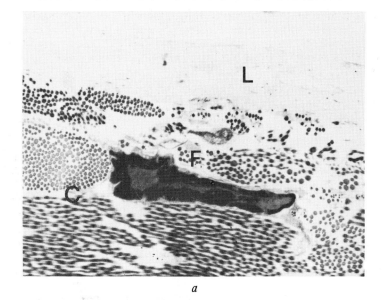

Fig. 1.9. Ultramicroscopic views of the structure of the normal condylar surface. L, Lamina splendens; F, Fibroblast; C, Collagen fibril bundles. *a,* Surface layers × 10560; *b,* At a lower level × 18200.

mucopolysaccharide and seems to bind the individual fibrils and their bundles, thus contributing to the total physical strength of the tissue.

Superficially, that is adjacent to the synovial cavity, there is a narrow zone of faintly fibrillar material which is more electron dense than the underlying ground substance (*Fig. 1.9a*). It varies between 1 and 2 μm in thickness and corresponds to the lamina splendens that is described in other joints.

ADAPTIVE CHANGES

The adaptive ability of the mandibular condyle has been mentioned earlier in this chapter. Throughout life it is constantly remodelling in response to changes in its functional environment, for example in compensating for worn or missing teeth. The process at a cellular level has been well described by Blackwood (1966a). He recognized three types of remodelling: progressive, regressive and peripheral. Peripheral remodelling results in the addition of tissue to the margins of the articular surface such as may be found in lipping or osteophyte production, but the most revealing observations are concerned with the progressive and regressive types.

In progressive remodelling there is proliferation and hypertrophy of the intermediate zone followed by an increased cartilage matrix production and an advance of mineralization into this newly formed tissue. The subarticular bony endplate is then established at a new level by osteoclastic resorption of the mineralized cartilage and its replacement by Haversian bone. In regressive remodelling, the process is reversed. First there is osteoclastic resorption of the subarticular bone and adjacent mineralized cartilage. The spaces left are filled by the proliferation of cells in the intermediate and remaining fibrocartilage zones.

It is of note that in each case the surface articular zone does not appear to be involved other than by passive adaptation to the changes that occur in the tissues beneath it. The structure of this layer remains remarkably constant, varying only marginally in thickness. This phenomenon has also been observed in other conditions affecting the growing condylar cartilage (Blackwood, 1962) and in animal studies (Blackwood, 1966b). It therefore seems probable that the fibrous articular zone functions principally as a protective covering, providing a smooth articular surface for the joint and not being generally involved or influenced by remodelling or metabolic changes.

These observations give rise to a fundamental concept in the understanding of mandibular joint problems. The mechanical changes in functional environment that result in articular remodelling, must be capable of being transmitted to the intermediate zone of cells and to the bone beneath, and not to be of sufficient magnitude to produce damage to the fibrous articular surface. In other words, the forces must remain within the physiological limits or functional capacity of the joint tissues. The balance is very fine and, as will be discussed in later chapters, degenerative changes in the joint occur when this functional capacity is either exceeded or reduced.

FUNCTIONAL ASPECTS

Normal joint function in such activities as chewing, swallowing and speech involves many complex mechanisms. It is not the purpose of this book to discuss these topics in detail, nor to become involved in such contentious issues as mandibular rest position and the various aspects of occlusion. The literature pertaining to these subjects is more than adequate and although an appreciation of the problem may be useful, a complete description here would in no way facilitate the understanding of temporomandibular joint disorders.

Certain functional aspects, however, are considered to be relevant and these are mandibular movement and the lubrication and load-bearing characteristics of the joint.

Mandibular Movement

Mandibular movement involves the co-ordinated relaxation and contraction of all the muscles of mastication. Each muscle pair may work synchronously, as in straight opening and closing, or individually as in side-to-side motion of the mandible.

The mandible is depressed by contraction of the inferior heads of the lateral pterygoids and, to a lesser extent, by the digastric and suprahyoid muscles. Elevation is through the action of the medial pterygoids, masseteric and temporal muscles. Lateral movements are executed by ipsilateral contraction of the temporal muscles with contralateral activity in both pterygoids.

Within each joint, jaw opening has two active components. Primarily there is a rotational hinge movement in the lower compartment. The second movement, the forward translation of the condyle, takes place in the upper compartment. Here the condyle moves downwards, towards and over the articular eminence. During horizontal sideways movement of the jaw, the ipsilateral condyle rotates with a slight lateral shift. This is known as the Bennett movement. There is a corresponding forward translation and rotation of the contralateral condyle.

Much of this description is based on electromyographical studies. Electromyography, however, does not distinguish between isometric contraction (when the muscle acts as a stabilizer) and isotonic contraction (when the muscle acts as a mover) (Ramfjord and Ash, 1971). Ricketts (1975) described the mandible as being slung in a complex web of muscles. Posture and movement of the jaw involve

16

very complex regulation of all the muscles in this web and thus they cannot simply be divided into agonistic and antagonistic groups.

Perhaps the most revealing electromyographical observation concerns the seemingly opposing actions of the superior and inferior heads of lateral pterygoid (Juniper, 1981). The superior head, attached to the meniscus, is inactive during opening while the inferior head, attached to the condyle, contracts. During normal closing and biting the superior head becomes active while the inferior head remains electromyographically silent (*Fig.* 1.10).

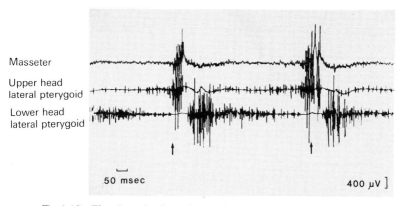

Masseter

Upper head
lateral pterygoid

Lower head
lateral pterygoid

50 msec

400 µV]

Fig. 1.10. The close-clench cycle. As the teeth occlude, indicated by the arrows, masseter and superior head of lateral pterygoid contract (upper two traces) while the inferior head relaxes (lower trace). The opposite occurs in the opening movement, again the two heads of lateral pterygoid act antagonistically. (Reproduced by permission of *Br. J. Oral Maxillofac Surg.*)

During normal opening the meniscus follows the condyle closely as it moves forward with the contraction of the inferior head of lateral pterygoid. The elastic superior lamella of the posterior attachment of the disc is stretched. On closing and clenching, when the inferior head is relaxed, the elastic recoil of the superior lamella together with the more rigid attachment of the inferior lamella, draws the meniscus backwards. It is postulated that the contracting superior head of lateral pterygoid holds the meniscus against the thicker bone of the articular eminence. Thus, this muscle acts as an important stabilizer of the temporomandibular joint.

The relationship of the meniscus to the condyle and temporal articulation during function is well illustrated in diagrams extrapolated from arthrographs in Chapter 4. These observations suggest that dysfunction occurs when the normal neuromuscular pattern is disturbed or when the working parts of the joint become damaged or deranged.

Lubrication

The normal free-sliding movement of the articular surfaces of the temporomandibular joint may be affected by:

  a. Instability of the meniscus, or

  b. A change in their frictional properties.

Failure of the joint ligaments and lateral pterygoid to co-ordinate and stabilize the meniscus will lead to incongruities between its shape and those of the joint surfaces. It may also allow its displacement or dislocation.

The low frictional properties of the joints are largely a function of the chemicophysical nature of the sliding surfaces and the interposed fluid film (boundary lubrication), the hydrodynamic lubricative property of the fluid playing only a secondary role. The physical condition related to this phenomenon might be likened to the difficulty of sliding two plain glass surfaces over one another even in the presence of abundant lubrication between them; if loads are excessive they begin to stick. The prevention of sticking of such congruous surfaces may be achieved, not merely by increasing the viscosity of the lubricating fluid, but by ensuring it has an affinity to each sliding surface. By virtue of such an affinity, a monomolecular film of lubricative fluid adheres to each surface and absorbs any free molecular activity which would otherwise be available to attract molecules on the opposing surface, and sliding takes place within this interface. Such boundary lubricant is specific for particular substances comprising sliding planes. Thus water or even glycerine is a poor lubricant for two glass surfaces, but a watery solution of oleic acid is a good one.

Boundary lubrication is probably not the only model to describe lubrication at every point of the articulating cycle. Depending on the relative motion of the surfaces, their relative geometry and applied load, other types such as hydrodynamic (full fluid film) and elastohydrodynamic (full fluid film accompanied by elastic deformation of the bearing surfaces) are probably relevant.

It follows, however, that any change in the structure of the articulating surfaces or of the quality or quantity of the lubricant is quite likely to bring about an alteration in the frictional characteristics of the joint.

Load-bearing Characteristics

In activities such as biting and clenching, forces generated by the masticatory muscles are applied across the teeth. The concept that these forces are also transmitted through the temporomandibular joint has been a controversial issue but its acceptance is vital to the understanding of both normal and abnormal function. Many authorities have contended that the joint is mechanically, anatomically and histologically unsuited to load bearing. More convincing evidence, however, has demonstrated that the opposite conclusion is the more likely.

Barbenel (1974) demonstrated in a theoretical study that the joint is load bearing during function and that the force across it during electromyographic analysis is at least 2·7 times the occlusal load. Similar observations have been made by Standlee, Caputo and Ralph (1977, 1979 and 1981). Using a model system they showed stress trajectories communicating with the condyle in both centric and excursive closing movements. The areas of major stress concentration corresponded to cortical and trabecular reinforcement within the human specimen from which the models were fabricated. Although its elliptical shape helped to reduce stress intensity, the condyle seemed better adapted to varied light forces rather than unidirectional severe, repeated forces.

This mechanical evidence is supported by the histological observations made earlier in this chapter. The increased thickness of fibrocartilage over the parts of the joint surfaces likely to bear the heaviest loads and the presence of elastic fibres, possibly to increase the resilience of those surfaces, seem to suggest that the joint is well adapted to resisting stress.

CHAPTER 2

THE COMMON DISORDERS

Successful management of a disease process involves both the establishment of an accurate diagnosis and an understanding of its aetiology in order that a rational treatment plan may be formulated. Many problems concerning the temporomandibular joint have been approached with an inadequate knowledge of either of these principles and treatment has been based solely upon empirical methods which have been judged by their capacity to work or not.

CLASSIFICATION

The classification that follows is by no means comprehensive but, for practical purposes, the problems that afflict the temporomandibular joint have been divided into common and rare disorders.

Common Disorders

1. Dysfunctions (TMJ pain-dysfunction syndrome, myofascial pain-dysfunction syndrome, etc.).
2. Internal joint derangements.
3. Degenerative disease (osteoarthrosis, ostearthritis, osteochondritis, osteoarthropathy).
4. Trauma
    a. Fracture.
    b. Dislocation.
    c. Traumatic arthritis, synovitis, etc.

Rare Disorders

1. Inflammatory
    a. Infection (following trauma, spread from middle ear or other adjacent structure).
    b. Rheumatoid arthritis (including juvenile chronic arthritis or Still's disease).
    c. Psoriatic arthritis.
    d. Crystal deposition diseases.
2. Ankylosis. Following trauma, infection, or other inflammatory conditions.
3. Congenital and Developmental. Defects such as those found in 1st and 2nd branchial arch syndromes, Pierre Robin and Treacher Collins syndromes: Hypoplasia, aplasia and hyperplasia of the mandibular condyle.
4. Neoplasia. Osteoma, chondroma, chondrosarcoma, secondary carcinoma.

It will be noted that rheumatoid arthritis is listed here as a rare disorder of the temporomandibular joint in spite of it being a relatively common disease. It has been shown that two-thirds of the patients suffering from rheumatoid arthritis have evidence of temporomandibular joint involvement (Ogus, 1975) but it only rarely presents in this site in the primary acute phase of the disease. Clinical and radiographical signs of involvement are found predominantly in the chronic phases and are probably indicative of secondary degenerative change. An explanation for this phenomenon will be described later in the chapter.

Fractures and dislocations of the temporomandibular joint are not considered in this book and for their management the reader is referred to an earlier handbook in this series, No. 5 *Fractures of the Mandible* by the late Professor H. C. Killey. Traumatic arthritis is almost always a temporary problem and may be the result of a direct or indirect blow to the joint causing damage to the articular surface or stretching the capsule or ligament. Even an anaesthetic intubation or a dental procedure can produce this problem. It is easily diagnosed from the history and if necessary treated, as with any other sprained joint, by rest and analgesics. Severe pain or disruption of the occlusion may necessitate complete immobilization of the mandible. The relevance of trauma to the joint in initiating or exacerbating a functional disorder will be discussed in Chapter 3.

The remaining common disorders, as described in the classification, are dysfunctions, derangements and degenerative disease. Generally these have been considered separately but it is likely that they have a related aetiology (Ogus, 1978; Schwartz and Kendrick, 1984) and it might be more logical to regard them as manifestations of a single problem. In pursuing the evidence for this argument, it is useful to review briefly the development of the concepts of pain-dysfunction syndrome and internal derangements, the pathogenesis of osteoarthrosis, and to compare certain epidemiological aspects.

PAIN-DYSFUNCTION SYNDROME

The beginnings of the temporomandibular joint saga have been traditionally attributed to Costen (1934) who described a syndrome of ten symptoms, ranging from neuralgia of the second and third divisions of the trigeminal nerve to tinnitus and altered sensation of the tongue and throat. He assumed that these apparently unrelated symptoms were due to the displacement of the condyle which compressed the Eustachian tube, the chorda tympani or the main trunk of the auriculo-temporal nerve, or eroded the glenoid fossa or the tympanic plate. The cause of the posterior displacement was said to be temporomandibular joint dysfunction consequent upon mandibular overclosure. Although these views were later considerably modified, they were the first to suggest a connection between malocclusion, mandibular dysfunction and facial pain.

The problems, however, may only be defined if there is some agreement between clinicians as to which group of symptoms should comprise the syndrome. It is complicated by the fact that in any particular case, the symptoms may change as the disorder progresses; even so, some attempt at a definition is reasonable and desirable. From the vast literature relating to the subject there now seems to be a consensus that the syndrome should be made up of one or more of the following:

    a. Joint clicking.
    b. Periodic inability to open the jaw fully (locking).
    c. Pain associated with the joint and the muscles of mastication.

The Occlusion

Following Costen's views, the occlusion became widely implicated as the principal factor in the establishment of a mandibular dysfunction. Management of the problem was therefore based on the analysis and treatment of such aspects as cuspal interference, occlusal dysharmony and overclosure. Indeed, it has been found that many patients improve under such a regime and its principles are still widely adopted in practice, based upon its success, possibly its strong suggestive power, and also the ready application of its mechanical techniques by dental surgeons who are well trained in the disciplines required in such treatment protocols.

Laskin (1969) put forward serious criticisms of these 'tooth theories'. He felt the explanations failed to show satisfactorily how occlusal interferences could develop in a functioning dentition unless they were iatrogenically induced. Neither did they show why most of the symptoms, particularly in the early phases of the condition, were related mainly to the masticatory musculature rather than to the joint itself. They also did not account for the high degree of clinical success in the treatment of such patients by different therapies, many of which did not alter the occlusion. Finally, and even more disconcerting for those who still held strongly to occlusal theories for the aetiology of pain-dysfunction syndrome, he showed that mock-equilibration (in which patients thought that their interdigitating dental patterns had been altered during treatment but, in fact, had not) produced as good results as when patients were treated by actual modifications of their occlusion (Goodman et al., 1976).

The Muscles

In the late 1950s, Schwartz and his co-workers recognized that there should be a shift of emphasis from consideration of occlusal factors to an understanding of the involvement of the masticatory musculature. According to Schwartz and Cobin (1975), pain in or near the joint is attributable to functional incoordination or dysharmony of the mandibular muscles and this idea gave rise to a new series of treatments including the use of exercises to correct abnormal jaw movements, heat and short-wave therapy to relieve muscle spasm and a variety of bite appliances, which possibly interfere with proprioceptive feedback from the dentition during function and thus allow re-coordination of the musculature. Again, all these treatments have proved helpful, which would seem to suggest that a disturbance in muscle activity might be the underlying cause of the problem. Further evidence for this view has been provided by Berry and Temm (1974) who measured and photographed infra-red emission from the cheeks. The masseter was found to be hotter on the affected side; the difference diminished during treatment and disappeared entirely when symptoms had ceased.

Much interest has been centred around the brief pause in electromyographical activity of the jaw closing muscles that occurs shortly after tooth contact in chewing. This is known as the silent period. Bessette et al. (1971) showed that the silent period of masseter activity in patients with the syndrome is longer than in persons with no symptoms. Beemsterboer et al. (1976) demonstrated that this electromyographical feature returns to within normal limits with bite appliance therapy.

The mechanisms whereby these changes in muscle activity arise, however, are still open to question. Yemm (1976) could find no clear evidence that malocclusion could lead to maintained muscle hyperactivity through the reflex mechanism in spite of the enormous weight of contemporary clinical opinion. There is, on the other hand, increasing evidence that hyperactivity of the jaw-closing muscles may originate in the central nervous system.

The Psyche

The existence of a psychological factor in the aetiology of many temporomandibular joint disorders is now well recognized and has led to hypotheses which largely implicate emotion, behaviour and personality as prime causes of pain-dysfunction syndrome.

Conversion Reactions

Classic Freudian psychology suggests that these joint problems may be conversion reactions. The mouth and associated musculature, on account of their expressive nature and possible erotic connotations, act as a focus for unresolved emotional and sexual tensions. These conflicts are thus discharged in the form of parafunctional oral habits as bruxism and other irrelevant muscle activity.

23

Personality Traits

Although endeavours have been made to uncover personality traits which could be correlated with pain-dysfunction patients, there is little convincing evidence that these people form a well-defined group (Rugh and Solberg, 1976). Personality traits are usually considered to be permanent but behaviour is also much influenced by short-term emotional states such as anxiety, hostility and anger. Many authorities have indeed confirmed that patients with temporomandibular joint problems are more anxious than control groups.

Emotion

Emotion is very frequently mirrored in an individual's face. Happiness, sadness, anxiety, frustration, fear and anger may all be registered by the muscles of facial expression and the closely related muscles of mastication.

It has been confirmed (Rugh and Solberg, 1976; Yemm, 1976) that patients with temporomandibular joint disease respond to emotional stress with increased activity in the masseter and temporal muscles. This might be in the form of excessive muscular tension or of parafunctional oromuscular activity.

The observations would certainly seem to support the psychophysiologic theory proposed by Laskin (1969). He suggested that masticatory muscle spasm is the primary factor responsible for the symptoms of pain-dysfunction syndrome. The most common cause was thought to be muscle fatigue produced by chronic oral habits that are often a tension-relieving mechanism.

Response Specificity

All individuals are subject to emotional stress, not only in exceptional circumstances but as part of everyday existence. Financial, personal and social problems are only three examples that affect everyone. Only a relatively small proportion of the population, however, has a temporomandibular joint disorder, and this leads to the concept of response specificity. Individuals may possess a specific physiological response to stressful situations and thus a parafunctional oral habit may simply be a particular person's mechanism for neutralizing these tensions.

The Joint

Taking into account the preceding arguments, it would seem reasonable to suppose that pain-dysfunction syndrome has a multifactorial aetiology. This is the most popular opinion and there can be little doubt that the occlusion, the musculature and the psyche are all involved to a greater or lesser extent; but this view hardly provides an explanation for so common a problem. Perhaps a more logical approach may be found when the joint itself is considered.

The temporomandibular joint is unique in many respects. However, in common with other synovial arthroses, proprioceptive nerve endings are found only in the sensitive tissue of the capsule and not in the fibrous articular surface, the fibrocartilage, disc or synovia. Hence, as Banks and Mackenzie (1975) have pointed out, it is quite probable that the pain of pain-dysfunction syndrome originates from within the joint as a result of pathological or mechanical deformation of the capsule. The additional reflex muscle spasm that this produces will, as in other joints in comparable circumstances, exacerbate the condition.

A great leap forward in the understanding of the basic nature of the problem has come with the advent of sophisticated radiographic techniques. Arthrography of the temporomandibular joint was first described by Nörgaard (1974) and the technique revised by Toller (1974c). However, in spite of a case described in the *Lancet* by Annadale (1887) internal derangement of the joint has been appreciated and accepted only very recently Farrar (1978) was the first to diagnose anterior displacement as a common cause of temporomandibular joint dysfunction. He and his colleagues instituted new lines of treatment based upon their findings and their techniques were soon followed by countless other researchers and clinicians. Thus many refinements to the imaging methods have been assessed, such as CT-assisted and videoscopic arthrography. The findings, however, only confirm the suspected malposition of the meniscus within the joint and that arthrography is a very useful diagnostic procedure for temporomandibular joint disorders.

The question, however, still remains. What causes the damage to the joint apparatus? It has been proposed (Toller, 1976) that it might occur as the result of repeated trauma, that is, repetitive overload. It has previously been difficult to accept this idea since it had been concluded that the temporomandibular joint has no load-bearing capacity. Mechanical and histological evidence now suggests quite the opposite and thus, if the joint is load bearing, it must, under certain conditions, be subject to overloading.

Repetitive overloading may result from increased muscle activity in the form of parafunctional mandibular movements. These are either reactions to stressful situations or, more probably, an individual's specific response in releasing emotional tension.

Further evidence for this hypothesis and the part played by other factors, such as occlusion, will be discussed later. The authors, however, believe the concept to be of vital importance in the understanding of temporomandibular joint disorders for it provides a basis for a logical explanation as to their aetiology and thus a rational approach to their management.

THE PATHOGENESIS OF OSTEOARTHROSIS

Although the pathogenesis of osteoarthrosis is still the subject of much research and debate, it has generally been agreed that the lesion is of a degenerative nature. Since it is a disorder associated with ageing, a 'wear and tear' explanation has been popular. Degenerative change, however, occurring in the joint of younger patients is not uncommon and individuals thought to be liable to osteoarthrosis by virtue of their occupations (professional footballers, pneumatic drillers and parachutists) have not been found to have a higher incidence of joint degeneration than the rest of the population (Editorial, *British Medical Journal,* 1977).

It now appears that cartilage is fatigue prone (Weightman et al., 1973) and thus a mechanical explanation is at present the most favoured. Repetitive overloading of a joint may lead to remodelling of the bone in the subchondral zone which may be detected radiographically by an increased bone density (sclerosis), an early sign of osteoarthrosis. This stiffened bone is not as effective a 'shock absorber' as before and hence there is an increased stress on the articular cartilage (Radin et al., 1972).

The function of cartilage in a joint is to act as a cushion. It consists of 70 per cent water (Muir et al., 1969) and when a load is applied the fluid pressure within the tissue rises, but water is driven out only slowly due to the proteoglycans which are hydrophilic and impede the flow of interstitial water as they are entrapped in the collagen network and remain within the cartilage (Freeman and Kempson, 1973). The water: proteoglycan:collagen relationship in cartilage is thus critical and any factor, be it traumatic or metabolic, which upsets the balance may initiate degenerative change.

This is only a very simplified view of the problem but it could be postulated that the degenerative process may be brought about either by an increase in the functional demands on essentially healthy tissue or by a deterioration in the functional capacity of the tissues themselves (Editorial, *Lancet,* 1973). In other words, as shown in *Fig.* 2.1, breakdown of the joint may occur when the tissues are subject to repetitive loading in excess of their functional capacity or when they are subject to normal loads where this functional capacity is reduced. The reduction is seen secondary to other diseases, e.g. rheumatoid arthritis, but it occurs most frequently as part of ageing. Muir (1977) has proposed that some persons have a genetic predisposition to osteoarthrosis in that they have lower levels of collagen in the superficial zone and are thus unable to withstand the stresses of impact loading as readily as those with higher levels.

The research that has led to these speculations has been concerned with the cartilaginous linings of the synovial joints associated with the

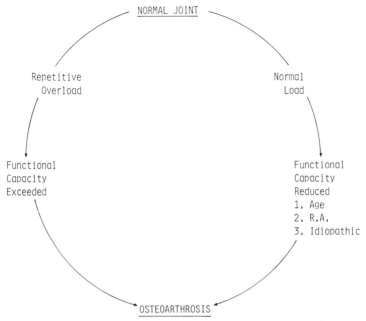

Fig. 2.1. The aetiology of osteoarthrosis.

long bones. It is assumed, therefore, that a comparable situation exists in the temporomandibular joint, albeit with a modified histological and biochemical picture.

EPIDEMIOLOGICAL COMPARISONS

Epidemiology has been described as the study of the distribution and determinants of disease frequency (MacMahon and Pugh, 1970). In other words, an epidemiological survey should not only estimate the distribution and frequency of a disease within the population, but also reveal factors that might be of significance in discovering its cause. Several such exercises have been attempted in relation to pain-dysfunction syndrome but a comparison is difficult as different diagnostic criteria and indices have been used. A study by Helkimo (1976) also highlighted another problem. Research on unselected populations has shown that symptoms of mandibular dysfunction are much more common than had previously been assumed. However, in the majority of these cases the findings are not subjective and a patient does not generally seek advice until there is pain or a relatively severe limitation of function.

Pain-dysfunction syndrome, as defined earlier in this chapter, is a worldwide problem more frequently encountered in countries or communities with advanced social systems. This has led to the suggestion that it might be related to neurotic tension. Helkimo's study found no great difference in the sex distribution of mandibular dysfunction but there can be no doubt that women predominate in any group of patients being treated for temporomandibular joint complaints. The ratio in various studies ranges from 3:1 to 9:1 and it is interesting to note that the figures are similar to those of patients attending their general practitioners or psychiatric clinics for treatment of neuroses. Weinburg (1977) has suggested that men have more non-oral tension-relieving mechanisms available to them than women have in our society.

Symptoms of pain-dysfunction are found in all age groups from the early teens to old age. Most studies indicate a peak incidence of between 20 and 30 years but this is not a consistent finding.

Epidemiological studies have also been carried out with regard to such factors as occlusion, personality and socio-economic status but the results are often contradictory. Few clear patterns have emerged although emotional tension and other psychic aspects are now probably the most frequently implicated.

There is again conflicting evidence as to how often degenerative change is found in the temporomandibular joint. Mayne and Hatch (1969) have stated that it is rarely seen. On the other hand Toller (1973) reported that in a study of 1573 patients with temporomandibular joint disorders, 130 (8 per cent) were diagnosed as having osteoarthrosis. Blackwood (1963) reported that arthritic changes were found in about 40 per cent of specimens from cadavers over the age of 40 (although not known to be clinically manifest previously), and Macalister (1954) found an even higher proportion of histologically abnormal joints from cadavers.

There are several possible explanations for these diverse findings. The condyle is continually remodelling throughout life, the amount and rate being mainly dependent upon functional changes. It is possible that many of the histological changes observed in the cadaver specimens, previously considered to be osteoarthrosis, were in fact due to remodelling associated with ageing or changes in dental state. Furthermore, the cadaver studies suggested that in the majority of cases, the degenerative disease first appeared on the posterosuperior aspect of the condyle. Clinical radiographs, on the other hand, usually reveal the anterosuperior aspect to be the most frequently affected and this is confirmed by postoperative condylectomy specimens. Blackwood's studies suggested, however, that the disease was often clinically silent and so its incidence in the population was higher than would seem by clinical observation.

Toller (1974b) felt that the reason why clinical osteoarthrosis of the temporomandibular joint had hitherto not been recognized was that

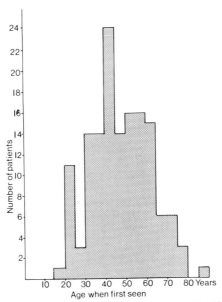

Fig. 2.2. Histogram illustrating the age range of 150 patients diagnosed as having mandibular osteoarthrosis.

the most important sign, the radiographically detectable erosion of the condyle, was not easy to detect on transcranial views, up until then the most frequently used projection for the study of the joint. With the transpharyngeal projection (Chapter 3) it is usually possible to achieve a finely defined image of the articular surface with minimal distortion and no overlying bony shadows.

The age distribution at first attendance of the 150 cases of mandibular osteoarthrosis described by Toller (1974b) is shown in *Fig.* 2.2. The mean age is 53 years but it should be noted that almost a third of the patients are under 40, a group that would normally be associated with pain-dysfunction syndrome.

In the same study it was found that females were affected six times as frequently as males. This is far different from the distribution found in generalized osteoarthrosis where the sex ratio is even, but it is of a similar order to that reported in pain-dysfunction syndrome.

A SINGLE PROBLEM

It should be apparent from the first two sections of this chapter that the authors believe repetitive overload to be the single underlying mechanism that is almost always responsible for dysfunction,

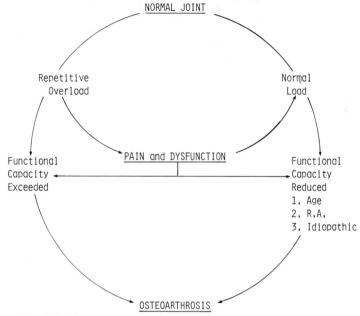

Fig. 2.3. The proposed relationship of pain and dysfunction to degenerative change in the temporomandibular joint.

derangement and degenerative change in the temporomandibular joint. Epidemiological comparison reveals that although pain-dysfunction syndrome tends to occur in a younger age group than degenerative disease, there is considerable overlap. Degenerative disease being more common in the older patient is merely an indication of the decline in the functional capacity of the joint tissues with age. Moreover, degenerative change in the temporomandibular joint, in common with dysfunction, is usually only active unilaterally.

The hypothesis is illustrated in *Fig.* 2.3. As stated earlier in this chapter, degenerative change may occur when the joint is subjected to repetitive overload in excess of its functional capacity or when it is subject to normal loads where the functional capacity is reduced. The initial reaction to the repetitive overload is frequently expressed clinically as clicking. This is the early sign of dysfunction and a reversible situation. Should the overload be relieved then the symptoms subside and function returns to normal. If, however, the overload should continue then the joint may lock and become painful. The joint becomes deranged and as the functional capacity of the tissues is exceeded degenerative changes take place. The evidence for these conclusions and a more detailed explanation is given in Chapter 5. From now on, therefore, the problem will be considered as a single disorder, mandibular stress syndrome. This title is not only illustrative of the increased stress upon the joint itself, but also of the most frequent aetiological factor, anxiety.

CHAPTER 3

THE CLINICAL EXAMINATION

There is little difficulty in diagnosing the majority of temporo-mandibular joint complaints as cases of mandibular stress syndrome, but before a treatment plan can be decided, it is necessary to establish the various aetiological factors. This involves a thorough and painstaking examination since many of the failures in the management of these conditions are due to a lack of diagnostic discrimination (Laskin, 1969).

Successful management is especially influenced by the doctor–patient relationship established at the first visit. The patient is therefore made to feel at ease as soon as possible, the consultation being carried out in a quiet and pleasant environment. An armchair in an office is far more relaxing than a dental chair in a treatment area full of equipment.

Anxiety is probably the most common aetiological factor and so, above all else, the patient requires constant reassurance that the problem is not serious and can be successfully treated. Early recognition of all aspects of the diagnosis, however, is rarely possible but, as the relationship between patient and clinician develops, the relevant information comes to light. It may thus be counter-productive to attempt the complete history, covering all the following aspects, at the first visit. Individual cases and circumstances vary widely and only experience will dictate to the clinician at what pace and depth it would be preferable to proceed.

HISTORY
Social and Occupational Information

An initial enquiry into the patient's social and occupational situation helps to establish an early rapport and may provide the clinician with valuable information. For example, there is the young housewife; not only does she have a husband, children and a home to care for but also the added stress of a part-time job. On the other hand an equally frequent visitor is the middle-aged housewife whose children have grown up and left home. She does not have enough to occupy herself.

A greater incidence of pain-dysfunction syndrome has been recorded among higher socio-economic groups (Rothwell, 1972). Thus, in many cases, it is the husband's occupation that is the more relevant.

The occupation, in certain circumstances, has a more direct influence on the joint. Telephonists, for example, may develop symptoms in the side to which they hold the telephone. A musical instrument player, continually posturing the mandible forward, may increase the load on the joint as do some singers with exaggerated mandibular movements.

Present Complaint

The complaint should be listened to with understanding. Although the clinician will have heard similar histories on many, many occasions, it is the sympathetic manner in which he reacts to the patient's own story that may be crucial to the outcome of the case. Again, the importance of the doctor—patient relationship at this stage cannot be overstated.

It is essential to record the symptoms accurately at the first visit as it is against these that the progress of treatment is evaluated. The patient should be asked if the condition is getting better or worse. Frequently there will have been a significant change between referral from one practitioner to another.

In order that the maximum amount of information may be gained from a temporomandibular joint history, it is preferable, as far as possible, to follow a set routine. In this way nothing is lost through neglecting to make the necessary enquiries. Individual clinicians will develop their own techniques but it is essential that the following points are always covered:

1. The nature of the symptoms.
2. When they began.
3. The precipitating factors.
4. The exacerbating factors, and
5. The pattern of the symptoms.

The majority of cases occur unilaterally although there may be a history of a similar problem in the contralateral joint which has resolved, with or without treatment.

The Nature of the Symptoms

The symptoms of a temporomandibular joint disorder may be recorded under the headings of pain, noises and dysfunctions.

Pain

Pain is the symptom that most frequently induces a patient to seek treatment. It is a subjective finding and thus difficult to evaluate. Individuals have differing thresholds and perceptions of pain and, in addition, there may be a psychogenic element.

The patient is asked to locate the discomfort and to indicate its spread. A finger is used to point to a specific site but if this is diffuse or vague, the palm of the hand may be used.

Numerous adjectives are used in describing the nature of the pain. Aching, stabbing, burning, gnawing, dull and sharp are a few; but the wide variation in individual tolerance and appreciation should be remembered. Excruciating to one person might well be a dull ache to another.

33

Common sites for the spread of pain from the joint are the ear, cheek and temporal regions; but, conversely, pain from adjacent areas may be referred to the joint. Sinus, ear and third molar problems especially must be ruled out. Temperature changes within the mouth giving rise to pain suggest that the origin is likely to be pulpal, which is often poorly located. Even sensitive tooth margins may give rise to referred pain.

Noises
The patient is asked to describe any noise that is heard in the joint. From the reply it is usually possible to assess whether this is basically clicking or crepitus. If it is not clear, a leading question must be asked; grating probably being the most descriptive adjective in this case.

Dysfunctions
Stiffness and locking are the two most frequent complaints of this nature, most other functional findings being signs and not symptoms. It is rare, for example, for a patient to remark that the jaw moves sideways on opening. Occasionally, a phrase such as 'my jaw feels out of place' is used.

Inability to occlude the teeth as normal, usually indicates an effusion into the joint or a traumatic injury and in these cases the complaint might be that the jaw feels swollen; but rarely is this apparent clinically.

The Onset of the Symptoms
The exact onset of the symptoms is often difficult to recall and the patient is only able to date with certainty recent acute attacks. It may be necessary to ask leading questions as certain symptoms, such as clicking, may be thought irrelevant although they may have been present for many years. The time scale is important for, as a rule, the shorter the history, the easier the disorder is to manage. Over a long period, more than one practitioner may have been consulted and such information may give some insight into the difficulties likely to be encountered in managing the case.

Precipitating Factors
In certain circumstances a precise history of the onset of the complaint is readily obtainable. Trauma, for example, may be related to a single blow or fall. A prolonged dental visit, removal of an impacted third molar or an uncomfortable high filling, may be remembered as events precipitating the complaint. More frequently, however, the onset was vague and insidious, although subsequently it may be recalled that the early symptoms coincided with a social or emotional upheaval.

Exacerbating Factors

Enquiries relating to the exacerbation of the symptoms may be the most revealing in the clinician's search for the underlying causes of the problem. Biting or chewing tough foods, opening the mouth widely while yawning or shouting and talking for long periods, are all examples of activities that aggravate the disorder.

Emotional factors, however, possibly have the greatest influence on the progress of most temporomandibular joint problems. A stressful situation such as an errant husband or boy-friend, redundancy or an examination, may be implicated. It is therefore wise, at this point, to make some gentle enquiry into the patient's personal background in order to reveal any anxiety or cause for emotional tension; but, as stated previously, it is unlikely that this information will be forthcoming at an early stage.

Bruxing or other habits are significantly common findings. The patient may be unaware of any of these until prompted but then realizes that, in certain situations, the teeth are clenched or some other irrelevant mandibular manoeuvre is made. These may occur in relaxed circumstances, such as sitting watching the television, and indeed nocturnal bruxism is a very frequent occurence. Clenching or grinding the teeth while asleep may exert a considerably greater load upon the joint system than can be achieved voluntarily while awake. Evidence for this observation may be obtained from the spouse or occasionally the parents who are able to hear the bruxing noises even through a closed bedroom door.

It is unusual for weather conditions to exacerbate temporomandibular joint disorders but a few patients complain that cold, wet conditions have an adverse effect upon their symptoms which improve in the summer months. This may be indicative of a chronic rheumatoid condition.

Recreational pursuits are occasionally implicated. Swimming or amateur operatics, for example, may require repetitive jaw postures that overload the joint. Wyke (1976) draws attention to a common (but often unrecognized) primary articular facial pain syndrome that occurs particularly (but not exclusively) in women in late adolescence or young adult life. He feels that this is due to the previous evening being spent in prolonged periods of intra-oral osculation, a common form of sexual play.

The Pattern of the Symptoms

Symptoms, especially pain, may be described as continuous, intermittent or occasional, but frequently a definite pattern emerges. A common finding is in a patient whose symptoms are minimal or even non-existent in the morning but, as the day progresses, pain and stiffness increase. Conversely there is the person who awakens with severe discomfort and unable to open the mouth. This condition, which subsides as the day passes, is usually an indication of nocturnal bruxism. Very occasionally, exacerbation of the symptoms may be associated with premenstrual tension.

Past Medical History

Although a concise medical history is necessary to establish the patient's general status, it should not be too searching at this stage as to cause concern that the condition may be a serious illness. On the other hand, an unrelated, underlying chronic medical condition may arouse anxiety that exacerbates the symptoms.

Certain aspects of the medical history are always important. Symptoms from other joints may indicate generalized osteoarthrosis or rheumatoid arthritis and even a family history of an arthropathy may be relevant. Medication, especially in the form of sedative or antidepressant, may indicate an underlying problem that the patient either does not wish to discuss or does not associate with the joint problems. A recent general anaesthetic may have been the precipitating factor, the mandible having been forced open in excess of its normal range.

Dental History

Situations where mandibular function may have been altered may be relevant to many temporomandibular joint conditions. Therefore factors that have interfered with normal biting or chewing habits should be recorded. Painful teeth and third molar problems are obvious examples, but prolonged orthodontic treatment may occasionally be implicated. Unsatisfactory dentures may also affect normal function and the clinician should be aware of the patient who wears his teeth for visiting and takes them out for eating.

The onset of symptoms is frequently preceded by a visit to the dentist, whether for a long session of conservation, the extraction of a difficult tooth or a general anaesthetic.

EXAMINATION

The clinical examination begins from the moment the patient enters the room. His general demeanour often gives some insight into his personality. He may be calm and lucid in his description of the symptoms or a nervous and poor historian. Anxious patients tend to fidget in their seats, play with their hands or shuffle their feet. Occasionally, parafunctional mandibular activity is immediately obvious. For example a patient may suck or chew on a lip, move the jaw from side to side or lean with his hand on the chin.

Any facial asymmetry may also be obvious at this stage.

Range of Movement

The patient is asked to open the mouth as widely as possible and, with the aid of a pair of callipers or dividers, the distance between the edges of the upper and lower incisors is measured. Nevakari (1960) reported that the mean value in males is 57·5mm and in females, 54mm. In his opinion, openings of less than 40mm in adults should be regarded as abnormal. Agerberg (1974) produced similar figures. The mean values were 58·6mm in males and 53·3mm in females. The lower limits were 42mm and 38mm respectively. However, it is important to take the depth of overbite into account. Mobility in the horizontal plane is measured by the shift in the incisal midline on extreme lateral excursions of the mandible to either side. Agerberg found that the lower limit for the normal range was 5mm in both sexes.

Deviation of the mandible during opening is noted. It may be towards or away from the affected side and associated with locking or pain. For example, the jaw will deviate towards the side of a locked joint indicating that in the affected condyle only the rotational componant of opening has occurred. The forward translation has failed. On the other hand, some patients appear to produce a click by swinging the jaw away from the affected side and back to the centre in a zig-zag manner as the mouth opens further.

Joint Noises

Clicking

Clicking is perhaps the most common of all temporomandibular joint complaints. This noise ranges from a soft, muffled thud to a loud, sharp crack but is rarely associated with any discomfort. It may take place early, midway or late in the opening movement.

A click may also occur during closing as well as opening and this has been termed 'reciprocal clicking' (Farrar, 1978).

A useful procedure at this stage is to test whether the dysfunction (i.e. clicking and/or deviation) is affected by opening the bite. The patient is asked to close the teeth while he or an assistant holds a pair of wooden tongue depressors between the molars on either side (*Fig.* 3.1). The clinician is then free to palpate the joints while the patient opens and closes the mouth. Abolition of a click with this test not only indicates that a bite appliance might be useful in the symptomatic management of the problem but also gives some clue as to the nature of the disorder. It would seem that, in this situation, the click has to be 'reloaded' by occlusion or near-occlusion of the teeth. The significance of this is discussed in the next chapter.

Crepitus

Crepitus is quite distinct from clicking. It is a grating or scratching sound occurring during mandibular movement, especially side-to-side

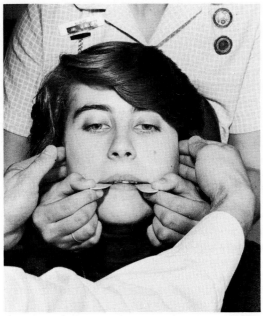

Fig. 3.1. Palpation of the mandibular joints with the patient biting on tongue depressors slid between the molar teeth (*see text*).

excursions. It is often better palpated than heard. Little or no additional information is gained with the use of a stethoscope in the examination of the joint noises.

Pain and Tenderness

Attempts by the patient or clinician to force open a 'locked' jaw are painful. The pain is felt in the joint and/or the associated musculature.

The joint and associated musculature are examined to elicit tender areas. Each joint is palpated gently while moving, from in front of the tragus and then just within the external auditory meatus.

The masseters and temporales, the superficial masticatory muscles, are easily palpated through the skin and scalp. The pterygoids, on the other hand, are only palpable intra-orally. The medial (internal) pterygoid is felt on the inner aspect of the mandibular ramus and the larger inferior head of the lateral (external) pterygoid, behind the maxillary tuberosity. Although some authorities recommend the palpation of the pterygoids, the present authors have not found that this provides any useful or reliable information. The examination itself is very uncomfortable and often causes the patient to gag.

With experience, the meticulous recording of many of the parameters of mandibular function is probably unnecessary. In practice, it is the diagnosis of a particular dysfunction that is the important factor and any measurement or other detail serves only as a basis for assessing the progress of treatment.

Intra-oral Examination

A full oral examination is carried out to assess the functional capacity of the dentition. This should include a search for any pathology that might be the cause of the symptoms, either on account of its nature or affect on mandibular function. A common example is an inflamed gum flap over a partially erupted third molar. The patient deviates the jaw to avoid biting this painful area. A periodontitic tooth or a high filling may cause a similar problem.

The following factors are then assessed:

1. Occlusal relationship.
2. Freeway space.
3. Overjet and overbite.
4. Missing teeth.
5. Prostheses, if present.
6. Attrition and wear facets, and
7. Premature tooth contacts.

Whenever the severity of the disorder renders functional assessment of the occlusion impossible, treatment is first started to obtain symptomatic relief. Analysis is completed later in the normal way. The authors, however, believe that although malocclusions may be involved in many temporomandibular joint problems, their role is generally secondary.

CHAPTER 4

RADIOGRAPHIC EVALUATION

James V. Manzione

Radiographic evaluation of the temporomandibular joint requires an understanding of its anatomy and function in normal and pathological states. Normal anatomy and function have been described in Chapter 1 and the controversies regarding the aetiology and pathogenesis of pain and dysfunction discussed in Chapter 2. It is becoming widely accepted that a large proportion of patients with temporomandibular joint problems have intra-articular abnormalities due to internal derangements and degenerative arthritis (Wilkes, 1978; Farrar and McCarty, 1979; Katzberg et al., 1980; Manzione et al., 1984b), the most common being an anteriorly displaced meniscus. In other patients, however, extra-articular factors may account for some or all of their symptoms. It is important therefore to identify internal derangements since different treatment modalities are employed if this intra-articular abnormality exists (Greene and Laskin, 1972; Farrar and McCarty, 1979; Goharian and Neff, 1980; Manzione et al., 1984c).

Although the main purpose of radiographic evaluation of the temporomandibular joint is to determine if an intra-articular abnormality is present, one must always consider the extra-articular causes of dysfunction. This chapter will (1) present and discuss the various temporomandibular joint imaging modalities and their radiographic interpretation, and (2) make recommendations regarding the selection and application of these radiographic techniques to identify and characterize intra-articular abnormalities in patients with temporomandibular joint dysfunction.

RADIOGRAPHIC TECHNIQUES

The superimposition of the bones at the base of the skull makes the temporomandibular joint a difficult structure to radiograph. Many conventional radiographic techniques have been described to overcome these difficulties (Blackman, 1963; Smith and Harris, 1970). Recently sophisticated techniques such as tomography, arthrography, computed tomography and magnetic resonance have become valuable, highly accurate methods of evaluating both bony and meniscus anatomy of the temporomandibular joint (Wilkes, 1978; Katzberg et al., 1980; Manzione et al., 1982; Helms et al., 1982; Manzione et al., 1984a;

40

Helms et al., 1984; Katzberg et al., 1985). Conventional radiographic techniques, however, still remain valuable screening methods to evaluate the osseous components of this joint. In a given patient comparing the radiographic image of the normal and symptomatic joint often helps distinguish pathology from normal variations.

Conventional Radiography

In clinical practice the transcranial and transpharyngeal projections are the most commonly used office techniques employed to evaluate the temporomandibular joint. Other views such as the submental vertex (SMV) or Towne's view may be obtained in certain situations. Each projection visualizes a particular aspect of the condyle and temporomandibular joint (*Table* 4.1). The choice of examination depends upon what information the clinician requires.

Table 4.1 Projection Selection for the Radiographic Examination of the Condyle

Condyle	Projection
Superior surface	Transcranial, transpharyngeal Towne's
Anterior and posterior surface	Transcranial, submental vertex (SMV)
Lateral and medial poles	Towne's, SMV
Joint space, glenoid fossa	Transcranial
Range of motion	Transcranial

Transcranial Projection

As the name implies, the transcranial projection involves the passage of the central X-ray beam through the cranium. There are many variations of the transcranial projection; however, the posterior auricuar approach described by Lindblom is preferred since it takes into account the long axis of the condyle.

1. The patient is seated upright with the head in the vertical position.
2. The film cassette is positioned in the sagittal plane on the side of the face over the joint of interest.
3. The X-ray tube is placed over the squamous portion of the contralateral temporal bone.
4. With the central ray entry point approximately 5 cm above and 2·5 cm posterior to the external auditory canal the tube is angled 20° anteriorly and approximately 20-25° caudally through the opposite condyle (*Fig.* 4.1).

The anterior angulation permits the X-ray beam to parallel the long axis of the condyle. The caudal angulation limits superimposition of the temporomandibular joint and ipsilateral petrous bones.

41

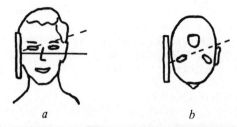

a   *b*

Fig. 4.1. Diagram illustrating the transcranial projection. Using the posterior auricular approach the central ray (dashed line) is angled 20–25° caudally (*a*), and 20° anteriorly (*b*) through the opposite condyle. The solid line represents the intercondylar axis.

The transcranial radiograph may be difficult to obtain in some patients due to variation in the relationship of the condyle to the bones of the skull base. Numerous head-holding devices have been reported to aid in performing the technique and in obtaining reproducible radiographs.

A transcranial series usually consists of views of each condyle in the closed mouth position (centre occlusion) and maximally open mouth position. If indicated, views at intermediate degrees of mouth opening can be obtained. Using this technique condylar shape, form, degree of translation and its relationship to the temporal bone can be assessed (*Fig.* 4.2).

Transpharyngeal Projection

Some clinicians prefer the transpharyngeal projection (*Fig.* 4.3) which is a technique based upon a description of McQueen (1937). It has been refined by Toller (1969) and the following account is yet a further development of the method.

1. The patient is seated upright with the head in the vertical position.
2. The teeth are separated approximately 2 cm by a bite-block. The separation of the teeth ensures that the condyle is advanced down the slope of the articular eminence, leaving the sheltering rim of the glenoid fossa. Owing to wide anatomical variation, it cannot always be ensured that the lateral rim of the fossa will avoid casting a shadow over the superior aspect of the condyle. However, in the majority of cases, this does not occur.
3. The film cassette is positioned over the joint to be radiographed. A useful guide is to place its posterosuperior corner just within the pinna of the ear. A soft wedge is positioned between the anterior part of the cassette and the patient's face (*Fig.* 4.4).

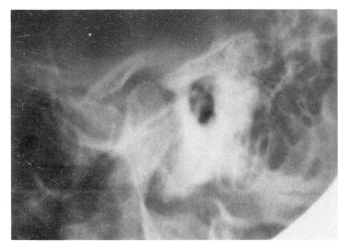

a

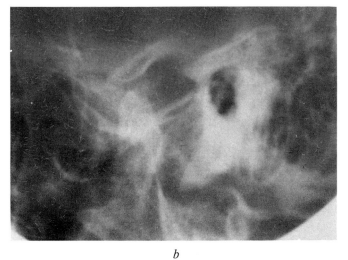

b

Fig. 4.2. Transcranial view of a normal temporomandibular joint. (*a*) closed mouth, (*b*) open mouth.

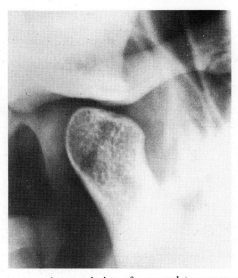

Fig. 4.3. A transpharyngeal view of a normal temporomandibular joint in a person aged 26.

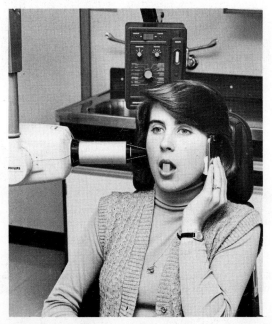

Fig. 4.4. The transpharyngeal projection. Position of the cassette and X-ray tube. The teeth are separated by about 2 cm.

4. The radiographic cone is positioned with its apex adjacent to the skin in a depression formed between the zygomatic arch above, and the sigmoid notch below. This may usually be palpated, especially in a thin-faced person. The tube is angled towards the condyle on the opposite side, that is 5–10° posteriorly and superiorly (*Fig.* 4.5).

The opening of the jaw allows passage of X-rays through the sigmoid notch, across the pharynx posterior to the pterygoid plates, and towards the medial aspect of the condyle on the opposite side. *Fig.* 4.6 demonstrates why this projection is frequently referred to as the 'keyhole' view.

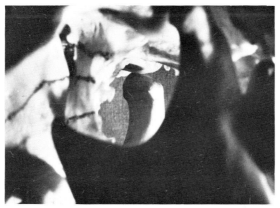

Fig. 4.5. Photograph illustrating the transpharyngeal projection 'keyhole view' on a dried skull.

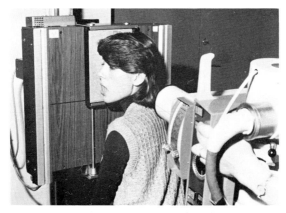

Fig. 4.6. The transpharyngeal projection in the radiology department.

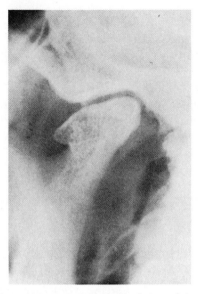

Fig. 4.7. Transpharyngeal view of a healed condyle following degenerative disease in a person aged 62.

The transpharyngeal view may be obtained with apparatus available
in a radiology department (*Fig.* 4.7). This technique is easier to adjust
and reproduce than with the dental cassette.

Transcranial v. Transpharyngeal

In the author's opinion, the transcranial projection is the single most
useful conventional radiograph since it demonstrates the condyle, joint
space, eminence, glenoid fossa and range of motion better than the
transpharyngeal which essentially only visualizes the condyle and
eminence.

The condyle is optimally seen on the transcranial projection since
(1) the central ray passes parallel to the long axis of the condyle and
eminence; (2) the caudal angulation of the central ray emphasizes the
lateral aspect of the condylar surface where the early changes of
degenerative arthritis have been reported (Katzberg et al., 1983a).
The projection is less sensitive to irregularities of central and medial
condylar surfaces.

The transpharyngeal projection produces an off-axis image of the
condyle and eminence. This results in a distorted view of the joint;
however, some clinicians believe this projection emphasizes the lateral
pole of the condyle. This projection is useful in detecting fractures of
the condylar neck and gross morphological changes of the condylar

surface. The transpharyngeal does not access joint space, the anterior aspect of the condyle or condylar motion, and may be difficult to obtain in patients with limited condylar mobility.

Due to variations in joint morphology and the relationship of the temporomandibular joint to the bones of the skull base one technique may provide a better view of the condyle than the other in a given patient. In certain patients neither method will adequately examine the joint. In these cases, and in situations when there is questionable or unclear findings on the conventional radiographs, or when more detailed information is needed, plain tomography or computed tomography should be performed to evaluate the osseous structure. These techniques are the optimal methods to evaluate bony morphology and will be discussed below. Many studies have demonstrated tomography to be more sensitive for detecting bony abnormalities than conventional radiographs (Stanson and Baker, 1976; Katzberg et al., 1980; Katzberg et al., 1983a).

Panoramic Radiography

Panoramic radiographic techniques will demonstrate both condyles on the same film. The axial inclination of the condyle as well as overlap of the condyle and glenoid fossa limit visualization of the condylar surface. On open mouth views overlap is decreased. Although a variety of special positioning techniques have been reported to improve condylar visualization, consistently good results may be difficult to obtain.

Tomography

Tomography is a precise radiographic method of evaluating the osseous components of the temporomandibular joint. Although there are several different tomographic techniques all utilize the basic principle of obscuration of the overlying structures by motion (Littleton, 1976; Stanson and Baker, 1976). The film and tube are linked to one another by a system of levers and then rotated around a point which is on the plane of the object being radiographed. The objects outside the plane are blurred by the motion while those within produce a sharp image. Complex motion tomography provides better image definition than linear tomography.

Although tomographic sections through the temporomandibular joint can be performed in many planes the lateral or sagittal section optimally visualizes the condyle, joint space, glenoid fossa and eminence (*Figs.* 4.8, 4.9). Lateral tomographic sections through the temporomandibular joint should be made perpendicular to the long axis of the condyle. This is accomplished by rotating the patient's head approximately 20° toward the side being examined (Coin, 1974). Contiguous tomographic sections made through the medial, central and lateral

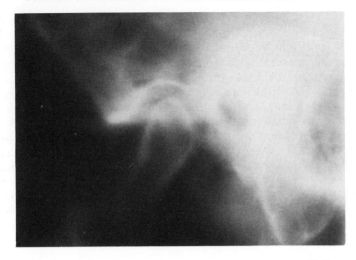

Fig. 4.8. Lateral plain tomogram of a normal temporomandibular joint.

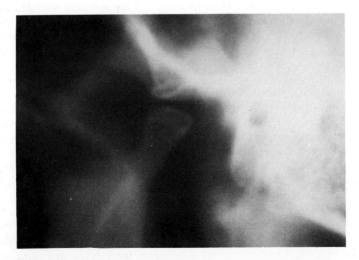

Fig. 4.9. Lateral plain tomogram of the temporomandibular joint demonstrating flattening and deformity of the condylar head.

portions of the temporomandibular joint permit a detailed evaluation of the condylar and temporal bone surfaces. Lateral tomograms are made with the mouth closed and selected views made with the mouth open. Tomograms made in the coronal plane are occasionally employed and when performed compensation for the angulation of the condylar axis should be made. Coronal sections are useful to evaluate abnormalities of the medial and lateral poles.

Although plane tomography is a clearly superior method than conventional radiographs for evaluating the osseous structures of the temporomandibular joint it does not evaluate the intra- and extra-articular soft tissues (i.e. meniscus and pterygoid musculature). Arthrography and, more recently, computed tomography and magnetic resonance are the only precise methods to determine meniscus configuration, function and position (Wilkes, 1978; Farrar and McCarthy, 1979; Katzberg et al., 1980; Manzione et al., 1982; Helms et al., 1982; Manzione et al., 1984a; Helms et al., 1984; Katzberg et al., 1985).

Arthrography

Temporomandibular joint arthrography has significantly improved our knowledge and understanding of condylar and meniscus relationships in normal and abnormal functional states (Nörgaard, 1947; Toller, 1974c; Wilkes, 1978; Farrar and McCarty, 1979; Katzberg et al., 1980; Manzione et al., 1984d). Until recently, arthrography has provided the only objective means of determining the presence of internal meniscal derangements in patients with temporomandibular joint dysfunction. It has become a valuable tool in distinguishing intra-articular causes (internal derangements) from extra-articular aetiologies of temporomandibular joint dysfunction particularly when plane films are normal (Katzberg et al., 1980).

Arthrography should only be performed in those patients who have pain associated with symptoms of dysfunction such as clicking or locking, especially in patients whose symptoms persist or are unresponsive to conservative symptomatic therapy. Generally, it is only necessary to inject the lower joint space with contrast though both spaces may be opacified. Injection of the lower joint space can be accomplished with a 23 gauge needle/catheter under local anaesthesia (Katzberg et al., 1980). Meglumine or sodium diatrizoate — 60% contrast materials are preferred and manufactured under a variety of names. Needle insertion and contrast injection is done under fluoroscopic guidance. Once the joint space is opacified the relationship of the condyle and meniscus is observed under fluoroscopy and recorded on video tape during mouth opening and closing. Radiographs are made in the open and closed mouth positions.

Normally the meniscus is observed on the surface of the condyle in both the closed and open mouth position (*Fig.* 4.10). If a click is

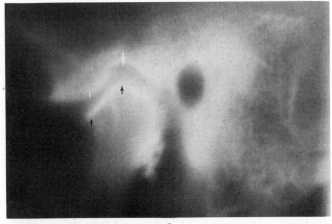

a

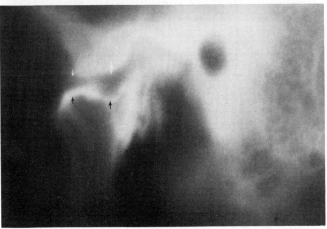

b

Fig. 4.10. Normal temporomandibular joint arthrogram. *a*, Contrast in the lower joint space (*black arrows*) outlines the superior surface of the condyle and the lower surface of the meniscus. The meniscus is the biconcave lucency between the contrast and temporal bone (*white arrows*). The anterior portion of the lower joint space (anterior recess) is tear drop in form (*small black arrow*). It delineates the anterior portion (band) of the meniscus (*small white arrow*). The posterior portion of the lower joint space (posterior recess) is convex in form (*large black arrow*). It delineates the posterior band of the meniscus (*large white arrow*). *b*, When the mouth is open the posterior band of the meniscus (*large white arrow*) creates a concavity in the posterior recess of the lower joint space (*large black arrow*). The anterior band of the meniscus (*small white arrow*) is outlined by contrast in the anterior recess (*small black arrow*).

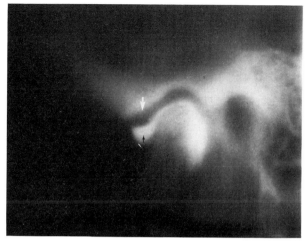

a

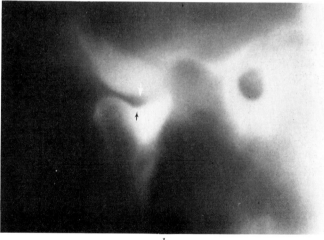

b

Fig. 4.11. Meniscus displacement with reduction. *a,* When the meniscus is anteriorly displaced the anterior recess is elongated and has a concave upper margin (*black arrow*) that is created by the anteriorly displaced posterior band of the meniscus (*white arrow*). *b,* At the time of the clinical click the meniscus slips onto the surface of the condyle. Once this occurs the arthrogram assumes a normal configuration. Compare with *Fig.* 4.10*b.* Note the concavity created in the posterior recess (*black arrow*) by the posterior band of the meniscus (*white arrow*).

51

present clinically or observed fluoroscopically spot films are made immediately before and after the click occurs (*Fig.* 4.11). This will distinguish clicking secondary to an internal derangement (meniscus displacement with reduction) from other sources of joint noises. In cases of meniscus displacement with reduction, these techniques will determine if the meniscus reduces in the early or late phase of mouth opening. In general, the earlier the meniscus reduces during translation the better the prognosis for conservative treatment. *Fig.* 4.12 is an example of the arthrographic findings of an anteriorly displaced meniscus in which reduction does not occur.

Other uses of arthrography include (1) determining if a perforation of the meniscus or posterior attachment exists, (2) the evaluation of splint therapy (Manzione et al., 1984c), (3) identification of loose bodies (Anderson, 1984), (4) postoperative evaluation in some cases.

Contraindications to arthrography include (1) infection of the overlying skin, (2) prior history of allergy to contrast material, (3) bleeding diathesis or anticoagulant therapy.

Computed Tomography

Arthrography is an invasive procedure that may be painful and at times difficult to perform. Computed tomography (CT) has been shown to be a useful non-invasive means of evaluating internal derangements and arthritis of the temporomandibular joint (Manzione et al., 1982; Helms et al., 1982; Manzione et al., 1984a; Sartoris et al., 1984; Thompson et al., 1984). CT evaluation of the temporomandibular joint does not require intra-articular or intravenous contrast material. Unlike arthrography CT provides not only detailed information regarding meniscus position and function but also provides information regarding bone detail. This is accomplished by selecting, via a computer, soft tissue and bone settings of each image.

Fig. 4.13 is a CT scan of a normal temporomandibular joint. The meniscus is on the condylar surface in both the closed and open mouth position. The low density (black) area anterior to the meniscus represents the lateral pterygoid fat pad (Manzione et al., 1984a). *Figs.* 4.14 and 4.15 are CT examples of internal derangements. In contrast to the normal joint, the anteriorly displaced meniscus is seen as a high density area anterior to the condyle. The displaced meniscus displaces the lateral pterygoid fat pad anteriorly (*Figs.* 4.14 and 4.15). *Fig.* 4.16 is a CT scan made at a bone setting. In this normal example the condylar surface is smooth and uniform. *Fig.* 4.17 is a CT example of degenerative arthritis.

The ability of CT to image the meniscus and osseous structures of the joint eliminates the need for conventional films, arthrography, and plane tomography in many patients. Assuming proper scanning technique, CT will demonstrate bone detail in virtually all patients;

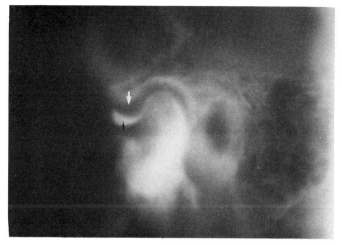

a

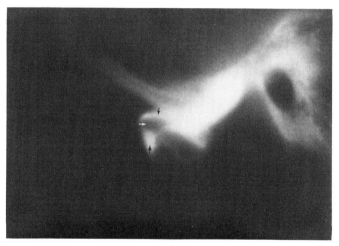

b

Fig. 4.12. Meniscus displacement without reduction. *a,* The anterior recess of the lower joint space (*black arrow*) is elongated and has a concave upper margin created by the posterior band of the displaced meniscus (*white arrow*). Despite attempts at mouth opening the meniscus remains persistently anteriorly displaced limiting condylar motion. *b,* If perforation of the meniscus or posterior attachment occurs contrast injected into the lower joint space (*lower black arrow*) will flow into the upper joint space (*upper black arrow*). The meniscus is the lucency between the joint spaces (*white arrow*).

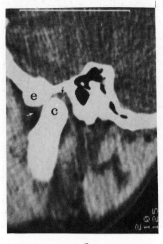

a

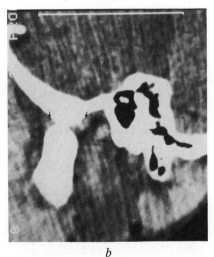

b

Fig. 4.13. Sagittal CT scan of a normal temporomandibular joint. *a*, When the mouth is closed the condyle (c) sits in the glenoid fossa. The meniscus is represented as a soft-tissue (grey) density between the condyle and glenoid fossa (*black arrow*). The lateral pterygoid fat pad (*white arrow*) normally is located within the angle formed by the articular eminence (e) and the condyle. *b*, On the open mouth view the condyle has translated to approximately the mid-portion of the eminence. The meniscus is the biconcave soft-tissue density between the eminence and condyle (*black arrows*).

54

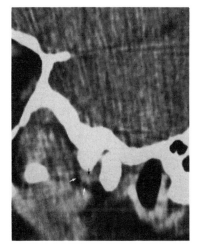

a

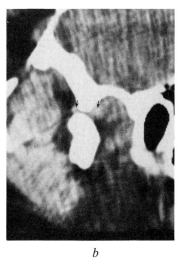

b

Fig. 4.14. Meniscus displacement with reduction. *a,* The anteriorly displaced meniscus is represented by the large soft-tissue density (*black arrow*) located in the angle formed by the eminence and anterior aspect of the condyle. The displaced meniscus pushes the lateral pterygoid fat pad, which normally sits within this angle, anteriorly (*white arrows*). *b,* Following the clinical click, when meniscus reduction occurs, the meniscus is seen in a normal position on the surface of the condyle (*black arrows*).

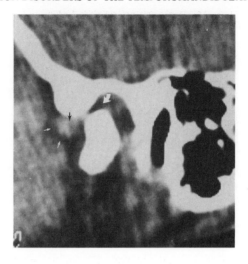

Fig. 4.15. Meniscus displacement without reduction. Despite attempts at mouth opening the meniscus (*black arrow*) remains anteriorly displaced. The displaced fat pad (*white arrows*) highlights the meniscus. In contrast to the normal joint (*Fig.* 4.13) no soft-tissue density is located between the condyle and fossa (*curved arrow*).

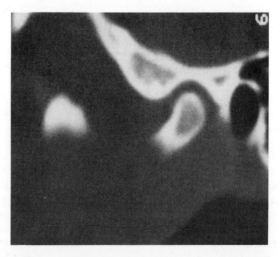

Fig. 4.16. Bone setting of a normal temporomandibular joint. CT images can be viewed at settings that optimize bone detail.

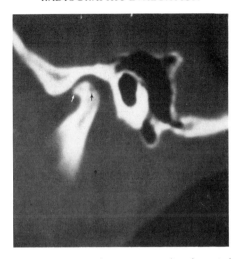

Fig. 4.17. CT bone setting demonstrates sclerosis, anterior lipping (*white arrow*) and cystic changes (*black arrow*) of the condylar head.

however, in approximately 10–15 per cent of patients CT will not adequately identify the meniscus and in such cases arthrography should be performed (Manzione et al., 1984a). CT images scanned directly in the sagittal plane are preferred to sagittal images reconstructed from axial scans due to their higher resolution and less radiation exposure.

The resolution of current CT scanners permits identification of degenerative changes within the meniscus, i.e. abnormalities in size, shape, position and the presence of meniscal calcifications (*Fig.* 4.18).

A disadvantage of CT compared to arthrography is that CT is less able to study the dynamics of meniscus function. CT can not detect perforations of the meniscus and posterior attachment.

Magnetic Resonance
Magnetic resonance first described in 1946 (Bloch et al., Purcell et al.), has been used primarily by physicists and chemists for spectroscopy. In the early 1970s (Lauterber, 1973) reports emerged demonstrating that magnetic resonance could be used to generate images. Magnetic resonance imaging (MRI) has been subsequently applied to obtaining physiological and anatomical information of body parts, particularly the brain and spinal cord. Recent reports suggest a role of MRI for imaging other body parts including the temporomandibular joint

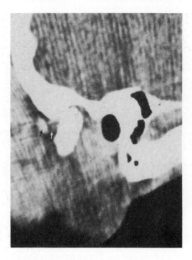

Fig. 4.18. Degenerative meniscus changes. The large calcification (*black arrow*) within the anterior portion of the displaced meniscus (*white arrow*) indicates that the meniscus has undergone significant soft-tissue degeneration.

(Helms et al., 1984; Katzberg et al., 1985). One of the main advantages of MRI over CT and other radiographic techniques is the absence of radiation exposure.

Magnetic resonance imaging is not dependent on differences in electron density (as conventional radiography and CT) but on proton density, tissue magnetic relaxation characteristics (T_1, T_2) and proton motion. The protons of the body (for our purposes hydrogen nuclei) are normally in a random state. Application of a magnetic field will cause the hydrogen nuclei to align themselves along the poles of the field. If a radiofrequency source is applied, the aligned nuclei will absorb energy and begin to resonate. If the original radiofrequency source is removed the nuclei will return to their original state giving off the energy they absorbed by emitting a second radiofrequency signal. The detection of the radiofrequency by a sophisticated antenna and processing of the signal by a computer will generate an image of the body based on differences in proton density (differences in proton density are primarily due to differences in water density).

Studies indicate that MRI has a potential place in temporomandibular imaging (*Figs.* 4.19 and 4.20) (Helms et al., 1984; Katzberg et al., 1985). Advantages of MRI are no radiation exposure and excellent soft-tissue imaging. Disadvantages include limited availability and high cost.

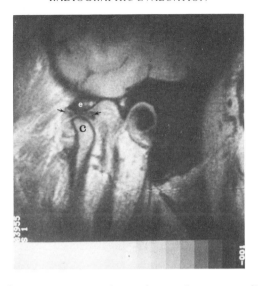

Fig. 4.19. Magnetic resonance image of a normal temporomandibular joint. Arrows highlight the normally positioned meniscus between the condyle (c) and the eminence (e). On magnetic resonance images cortical bone is black. (Courtesy of Richard W. Katzberg, University of Rochester, New York.)

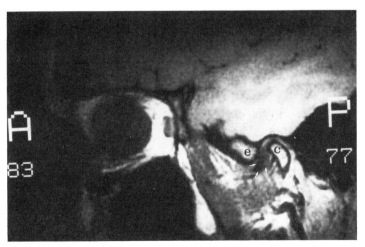

Fig. 4.20. Magnetic resonance image of anterior meniscus displacement. The displaced meniscus is represented by the black area (highlighted by *white arrows*) between the eminence (e) and the anterior aspect of the condyle (c). (Courtesy Richard W. Katzberg, University of Rochester, New York.)

RADIOGRAPHIC INTERPRETATION

As stated at the beginning of this chapter, the role of temporomandibular joint radiography is to determine if patients with temporomandibular joint pain and dysfunction have intra-articular abnormalities (internal derangements, degenerative arthritis) or extra-articular pathology. When selecting a radiographic procedure one must recognize its limitations. Identifying patients with intra-articular abnormalities on the basis of conventional radiographs alone is difficult. Normal conventional radiographs and even normal plain tomograms do not rule out the possibility of an intra-articular soft-tissue abnormality. In one study only 22 per cent of patients with internal derangements had evidence for degenerative arthritis on plain tomograms (Katzberg et al., 1983a). There are certain abnormalities on conventional radiographs and plain tomograms that correlate with the presence of internal derangements.

Joint Surface (Degenerative Arthritis)

The joint surface can be evaluated by conventional radiographs but is best visualized on plain tomograms or computed tomography. Although erosions of the joint surface on plain films are the earliest radiographic signs of an internal derangement, they occur late in the disease process (Toller, 1973). In patients with chronic clicking (symptoms of meniscus displacement with reduction) erosions may first appear on the posterior aspect of the condylar surface (Katzberg et al., 1983a). Erosions on the anterior and superior surface of the condyle are usually associated with anterior meniscus displacement without reduction (Katzberg et al., 1983a). As the derangement becomes more chronic distortion of condylar form, anterolateral osteophyte formation and sclerosis may occur. Flattening and degenerative changes involving the articular eminence is a late finding often associated with performation of the meniscus or posterior attachment.

Bone abnormalities of the temporomandibular joint are not specific for an internal derangement. A systemic inflammatory arthritis (i.e. rheumatoid arthritis, psoriatic arthritis), can affect the temporomandibular joint and result in erosions and secondary degenerative arthritis (Ogus, 1975). Degenerative changes of the temporomandibular joint in a patient without a history of a systemic arthritis strongly suggests an internal derangement; however, some patients in an older age group develop a primary degenerative arthritis with no meniscus abnormality. Bony changes are not very sensitive for internal derangements since they occur late in the disease process.

Joint Space and Condylar Position

This is perhaps the most controversial aspect of the radiological evaluation of the temporomandibular joint. The dimension of the radiological space between the inferior and superior articulating surfaces is difficult to assess and is probably only relevant if the finding is extreme in comparison to the contralateral joint. Many attempts have been made to standardize a technique whereby the joint space and condylar position can be measured in the hope that it would predict the presence of an internal derangement. The results are largely unpredictable and unreliable. Controversy still persists (Katzberg et al., 1983b; Weinberg, 1972; 1979; Farrar, 1978).

Joint Movement

Joint movement can be assessed clinically in many cases. If translation is limited the clinician must determine if extra-articular factors (i.e. muscle spasm) and/or intra-articular abnormalities (i.e. internal derangements, loose bodies, or degenerative arthritis) are the cause. In these patients, radiographic assessment can be helpful. Comparison of both sides is important in both the clinical and radiographic evaluation. In a patient with limited condylar translation, who has radiographic evidence of degenerative arthritis, an internal derangement is likely and further evaluation by arthrography or computed tomography should be considered. In patients with decreased translation who have no radiographic evidence of degenerative arthritis, an internal derangement cannot be excluded. If symptoms do not resolve following a short period of conservative treatment, an internal derangement should be suspected and further evaluation with arthrography or computed tomography considered. Some patients with meniscus displacement with reduction (clicking) have hypermobility of the condyle on the symptomatic side (Katzberg et al., 1982).

CONCLUSIONS AND PERSPECTIVE

Technology has presented the clinician with many sophisticated radiographic imaging modalities for the evaluation of the temporomandibular joint. Radiographic studies should be thought of as a diagnostic aid and not a substitute for good clinical judgement and experience. When and which imaging modality should be performed is controversial. The need for and the selection of radiographic techniques should be determined on an individual basis.

Conventional radiographs are helpful screening methods to evaluate the osseous components of the joint; the transcranial view is the most useful. Conventional radiographs aid in screening for arthritis, fractures, ankylosis, tumour, dislocations, hyperplasia, hypoplasia, and other osseous afflictions of the joint. Such abnormalities are better defined and evaluated by plain or computed tomography.

If degenerative arthritis is detected on conventional radiographs or tomography, and unusual causes of this condition are ruled out, an internal derangement can be considered likely. Normal conventional radiographs and plain tomograms, however, do not rule out the possibility of an internal derangement.

If there is a suggestion of an internal derangement clinically, on conventional films, or tomography, only arthrography, computed tomography or magnetic resonance can definitively establish the diagnosis and determine the extent of the intra-articular abnormality and degree of meniscus dysfunction and degeneration.

It is not possible nor necessarily desirable to obtain these sophisticated radiographic techniques in all patients with temporomandibular joint symptoms. Many patients respond quite readily to conservative symptomatic therapy. Those patients who do not readily respond or have an unclear clinical picture would benefit from an arthrogram or CT scan whichever is available and performed well in a given community.

The relative advantage of computed tomography and arthrography have already been discussed. Magnetic resonance is a desirable imaging modality since there is no radiation exposure to the patient. Preliminary work suggests it is a promising method for detecting internal derangements. Unfortunately, its availability is limited and its cost high. A future role of current imaging modalities, that has just begun to be utilized, is the use of these studies to assess clinical and surgical treatment. Such studies should certainly re-evaluate our current treatment modalities and better establish the indications, timing and selection of diagnostic imaging procedures.

CHAPTER 5

MANDIBULAR STRESS SYNDROME

Mandibular stress syndrome is a disorder generally confined to highly developed communities and thus most frequently associated with neurotic tension and emotional stress. It is difficult to assess its incidence other than to concede that it is an exceedingly common problem. Boering (1966) reported that at least one of the main symptoms of clicking, stiffness and pain had been experienced by approximately one-fifth of the population by the age of 30. Indeed, objective studies of unselected groups reveal that mandibular dysfunction is even more widespread (Helkimo, 1976).

Most mandibular dysfunctions, however, do not give rise to symptoms and, even when they do, individual tolerance varies widely. Some patients present early with a complaint, while others wait many months or years before seeking advice. Many have recurrent bouts of trouble but it is only when they suffer an acute episode or the condition begins to interfere with everyday life, that they require treatment.

The age distribution is wide. Teenagers are seen as frequently as patients in their sixth and seventh decades. Although Helkimo could find no great difference in the frequency of dysfunction between the sexes, females dominate actual patient studies, the reported ratios ranging from 3 : 1 to 9 : 1.

AETIOLOGY

Underlying Cause

The underlying cause of mandibular stress syndrome may be regarded as the emotional stress and tension to which our modern society subjects us daily. Although tolerance and reaction to these stimuli vary enormously, some people, in attempting to neutralize their effects, develop specific physiological responses. One such response is *parafunctional mandibular activity* which generally takes the form of bruxism or another oromuscular habit.

The repetitive impact of the muscular forces, acting through the mandible, overloads the joint and results in the characteristic features of pain and dysfunction. In certain circumstances the disorder may progress and degenerative change occurs.

Predisposing Factors

Certain other factors may influence the overload. Malocclusions, masticatory inefficiencies and trauma initiate, modify or exacerbate the problem but it would seem unlikely that any one is a cause in itself.

There is the clinical impression, for example, that a disproportionate number of patients with Angle's Class II, division 2 malocclusions suffer from the disorder. A similar group is composed of individuals who lack satisfactory posterior occlusal support. Berry and Watkinson (1978) have attributed these observations to the incisor relationship. During the initial stage of opening, the condylar movement is almost pure rotation. The excessive degree of this component, necessitated by the deep overbite, stretches the upper head of the lateral pterygoid muscle leading to failure of its stabilizing action on the disc, which may slip laterally, producing a click.

The main problem with such an explanation is that it does not account for the majority of people with these particular occlusal derangements and inadequacies who function quite normally without symptoms. Banks and Mackenzie (1975) have suggested that situations such as loss of molar support or change in the vertical dimension of the bite, alter the theoretical directions of the forces acting on the mandible and consequently the load operating through the condylar head. They are thus predisposing factors, rendering the joint more susceptible to overload.

A traumatic incident may precipitate a disorder by damaging the articular surface, capsule or ligaments. Examples are a direct or indirect blow to the joint, excessive stretching during a dental extraction or an anaesthetic, or a rapid change in the occlusion following a conservative or prosthetic procedure.

CLINICAL FEATURES

The patient with mandibular stress syndrome presents with one or a combination of the following clinical features:
1. Pain and/or tenderness over the joint.
2. Joint noises.
3. Altered mandibular function.

Most cases are unilateral, possibly because the majority of the population possess a dominant chewing or functional side.

The various signs and symptoms have been described in the clinical examination. It is the combination of these features that enables the diagnosis and staging of the disorder to be made.

Early Disorder

A single click is the most common joint noise and, early in the disorder, occurs quite painlessly and usually without noticeable deviation of the jaw. It may present at the beginning of the opening movement, when it can be abolished by opening the bite a few millimetres, or at some point later in the cycle.

This may be the only clinical sign of a disorder for a long period and, especially if it is only a soft click, give rise to little concern or inconvenience. A louder and more pronounced click, however, may prove embarrassing.

Intermediate Signs

Simple clicking may continue for many years before progressive discomfort forces the patient to seek advice. This may be joint stiffness, or pain on biting and wide opening. The joint and associated musculature become tender to palpation. Later there may be increasing difficulty in opening the mouth widely. The joint may click on both opening and closing and in doing so, the jaw deviates away from and then back to the affected side in a seemingly laboured fashion. It is as though the patient consciously has to unlock the joint before being able to open the mouth to its full extent.

The jaw now may lock completely. This occurs at the point where the joint would have clicked were the patient able to open the mouth fully. The chin deviates towards the affected side and attempts to open the jaw more widely are quite painful. No forward translation of the joint occurs on the affected side.

The order of the above two stages, however, is inconsistent. There may be periods when the joint is locked completely and times when, by manoeuvring the jaw sideways, the patient is able to unlock and continue opening. A large proportion of patients awake in the morning with a very stiff or locked jaw. This suggests a nocturnal bruxing habit. Others are almost symptom-free at the beginning of the day but gradually, towards evening, stiffness and pain develop.

Late Changes

Crepitus, described by the patient as grating or crunching, is indicative of degenerative change. Usually it is found in patients with a long history of a temporomandibular joint disorder but occasionally, even in the younger patient, it may occur within a few months of the initial symptoms. Alternatively, in the older age group, it may present as the primary symptom. The most consistent method of eliciting this clinical feature is to ask the patient to move the jaw from side to side. Crepitus often is palpated more easily than heard.

Pain, tenderness and stiffness may or may not be associated with crepitus, but where crepitus follows a long history of painful locking, the jaw gradually may become easier to move.

It would simplify the diagnosis of mandibular stress syndrome if the above order of clinical features could be ascribed to each case of the disorder. Frequently the signs and symptoms do not follow any particular pattern. For example, multiple clicks may occur at the same time as crepitus and, in spite of greatly altered functional patterns, there may be little pain. However, bearing in mind these limitations, the above description, together with relevant radiographic information, is a useful guide in diagnosing the disorder.

RADIOGRAPHIC FINDINGS

Using conventional techniques the majority of patients with mandibular stress syndrome have no radiographically detectable lesions. Evaluation of the joint space may suggest an internal derangement but generally the only definitive findings are degenerative change. Signs of this are found in about 8 per cent of cases (Toller, 1973) but are not always detectable at the first visit. They are usually visible only on the condylar surface although it seems likely that they occur just as frequently on the temporal articulation which is more difficult to demonstrate radiographically.

A quite definite radiographic sequence occurs (*Figs.* 5.1, 5.2). Initially there is a simple loss of density of the condylar surface, opposite the principal point of articular contact, at the anterosuperior aspect, or just behind. Soon a rough or woolly appearance develops with a

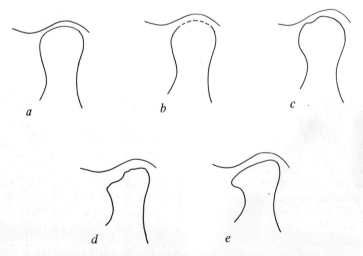

Fig. 5.1. Diagram illustrating the typical progression of a degenerative lesion in the condyle (drawn from radiographs): *a*, Normal; *b*, Loss of cortical outline; *c*, Erosion; *d*, Destruction and *e*, Remodelling.

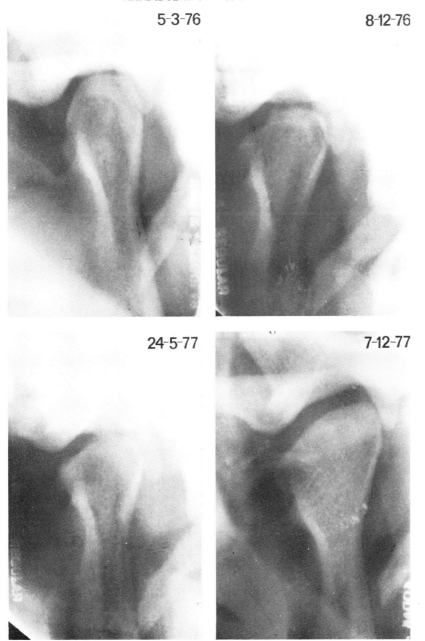

Fig. 5.2. Radiographs illustrating the progression of an erosive lesion of the condyle in a 20-year-old male.

spreading rarefaction in the bone beneath the surface. The fully developed disease usually shows a saucer-shaped erosion or erosions which may heal or proceed further to a gross destruction of the normal condylar anatomy. Occasionally osteophytic 'lipping' may be observed at the anterior edge of the condyle (*Fig.* 5.3). The articular surface is now intact but the shape of the healed condyle may range from being only slightly flattened to being completely remodelled (*Fig.* 5.4).

The time scale of these changes generally varies with age. In young persons there may be only 6–9 months between the initial radiographic finding and the healed condyle. In older patients the changes may be spread over 2–3 years.

The radiographic findings from arthrography and computed tomography have been described in detail in the preceding chapter. There is no doubt that this information has been of vital importance in the understanding of temporomandibular joint disorders. It has enabled the researcher to view the meniscus in both normal and abnormal function. In the clinical situation it may confirm meniscal displacement or damage in a deranged joint (*Figs.* 4.11 – 4.14).

DIFFERENTIAL DIAGNOSIS

Made on the basis of the preceding clinical and radiographical findings, the diagnosis of mandibular stress syndrome is rarely difficult. Occasionally, however, the symptoms may be confused with dental pain, earache and the various facial neuralgias. If there is doubt these must be excluded.

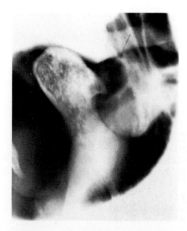

Fig. 5.3. Transpharyngeal radiograph showing an osteophyte at the anterior edge of the condyle.

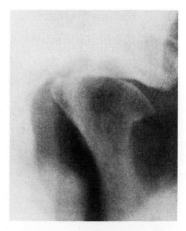

Fig. 5.4 Transpharyngeal radiograph of a remodelled condyle.

Traumatic synovitis and simple joint strain are usually related to a single episode and thus have an acute onset. Radiographs will rule out a fracture. In severe synovitis, normal intercuspation of the teeth, especially on the affected side, may be difficult due to joint effusion. Generally, although somewhat slowly, the problem is resolved with rest. Occasionally, on the other hand, it may progress to mandibular stress syndrome.

Rheumatoid arthritis may be ruled out, if suspected, by a normal erythrocyte sedimentation rate and negative serology. The disease, however, is rarely confined, if at all, to the temporomandibular joints. There is generally a polyarthritis and evidence of other systemic manifestations. In rheumatoid arthritis the temporomandibular joint is more likely to be affected bilaterally and erosions are frequently found elsewhere than the anterosuperior surface of the condyle (*Fig.* 5.5).

Several rare conditions may have to be excluded. An elongated styloid process, due to calcification of the stylohyoid ligament, is said to give rise to symptoms that may be confused with a temporomandibular joint problem (Eagle's syndrome). The patient also complains of the feeling of a foreign body in the throat. The tip of the process may be palpated in the tonsillar fossa and its length demonstrated radiographically on both lateral and postero-anterior projections.

Infective arthritis may be due to the spread of infection from adjacent structures or following trauma, or by the presence of a specific organism (e.g. gonococcus). Psoriatic arthritis may occur as a rare

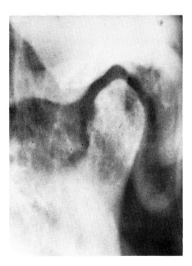

Fig. 5.5. Transpharyngeal radiograph illustrating an erosion of the anterior surface of the condyle in a 61-year-old female with rheumatoid arthritis.

reactionary inflammation of the joint in longstanding psoriasis of the skin. Finally, the severity and persistence of symptoms might suggest a secondary tumour deposit or, even more rarely, primary neoplasia.

SPECIAL INVESTIGATIONS

The preceding clinical, radiographic and aetiological accounts do not offer in themselves a satisfactory explanation of the pathophysiology of mandibular stress syndrome. Before suggesting an hypothesis it is useful to discuss the data obtained from the special investigations of histopathology, electron microscopy and electromyography.

Histopathology

It has generally been assumed that the condyles of patients suffering from pain and dysfunction of the temporomandibular joint have a normal appearance, at both macroscopic and microscopic levels. This was not so in the study described by Toller (1974a). All 10 cases were patients who had severe symptoms that failed to respond to the usual therapies. They were finally treated with conservative surgical procedures (capsular rearrangements). In some of the cases there were undulations of the condylar surface which suggested subarticular collapse. The occasional dullness of parts of the fibrous tissue covering of the articular surface suggested fibrillation, similar to that in early osteoarthrosis.

Histological examination has also been carried out on joints or joint surfaces removed from patients with both clinical and radiographical manifestations of degenerative change, the symptoms of which again were resistant to conservative therapy. Owing to the focal nature of the articular lesions and the frequent juxtaposition of degenerative and reparative processess occurring in a single joint at any particular time, difficulty in interpretation can easily arise. However, by studying sections from well documented cases, it has been possible to build up a histological picture of the process as it relates to the previously described course of symptoms and radiographical changes.

Fibrillation

The first indication of degenerative change generally occurs in the area of articular contact across which the greatest loads pass. There appears to be a progressive loss of cohesion between the bundles of collagen that make up the surface fibrous layer of the joint. Horizontal clefts, in which fluid collects, are formed between the bundles (*Fig. 5.6a*) which then fray off into the joint cavity (*Fig. 5.6b*).

With the fibrillation there is hypertrophy and increased mineralization of the subarticular cartilaginous zone. This results in a consolidation of the articular endplate which may extend down into the cancellous portion of the condyle, causing remodelling of the bony trabeculae, but leaving a normal bone marrow.

Denudation and Eburnation

With the gradual loss of all the fibrous tissue surface, there is a simultaneous maturation of the cartilage layer into a complete bony endplate.

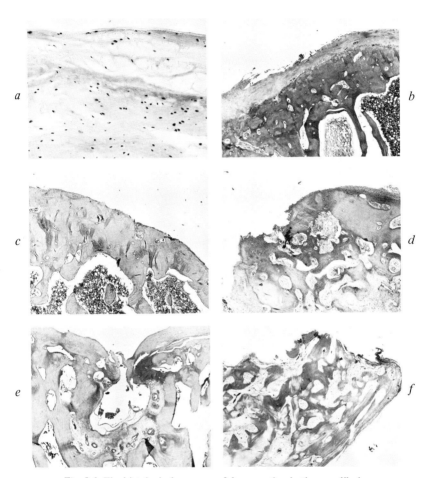

Fig. 5.6. The histological progress of degeneration in the mandibular condyle. *a*, Early interfibrillar degeneration of the articular surface over normal cartilage and bone. × 80. *b*, Fraying off of the fibrous articular surface into the lower joint compartment and a thickening of the bony endplate. × 12·5. *c*, The articular surface denuded of all fibrous layers but with a normal marrow beneath the bone. × 25. *d*, Perforation of the articular endplate and underlying fibrosis of the marrow. × 15. *e*, Cyst formation below an eroded articular surface. × 15. *f*, Gross erosive changes and replacement of all the marrow space with fibrous tissue. × 12·5.

The denuded surface (*Fig. 5.6c*) becomes denser and may appear 'worn' or 'polished', the process being termed 'eburnation'.

Perforation
Further progression of the lesion may occur as the endplate becomes thinned, defective and insufficient to shut off the articular cavity from contact with the bone marrow (*Fig. 5.6d*). This produces a fibrotic reaction within the cancellous spaces.

Subarticular Collapse
Occasionally small cysts occur in the bone deep to the eroded surface (*Fig. 5.6e*). They probably develop following degenerative change in the fibrous tissue that has come to occupy the marrow spaces in the subarticular bone. Later the cyst walls collapse giving way to generalized trabecular bone destruction.

Erosion
This stage involves the loss of more and more trabecular bone which results in a deepening of the lesion and a further replacement of the normal marrow spaces with fibrous tissue (*Fig. 5.6f*). There is widespread erosion of the condylar head and frequently gross destruction of the normal condylar anatomy.

Repair
No histological section has been seen in which the stage of massive erosion was followed by complete repair with reformation of a bony endplate. However, many radiographs have shown that this final clinically satisfactory situation does occur. It seems likely that a new fibrous articular surface develops from the synovial margins and that a new cortical endplate develops beneath it.

It must be noted, however, that healing may occur at *any* stage of the condition and that fibrillation does not inevitably progress to a gross destruction of the joint.

In general these histological changes are not dissimilar to those seen in degenerative disease in other joints. Differences are principally clinical and epidemiological but the most striking phenomena, related to the temporomandibular joints, are the rapid progress of the disorder and its tendency towards natural repair.

It is probable that these are due to the great remodelling potential of the joint. Indeed, in many cases, especially in younger patients, degeneration may be regarded as a rapid means of remodelling.

Electron Microscopy
The ultramicroscopic structure of the articular surface of the normal mandibular condyle has been described in Chapter 1. In order to observe

changes in abnormal condyles, biopsy specimens have been obtained from:

a. Cases of severe pain and dysfunction of the temporomandibular joint which have not responded to the usual therapies and have been treated by a conservative procedure (Toller, 1977a), and

b. Cases with clinical and radiographic evidence of degenerative change which again have failed to respond to routine measures and have been treated by surgical excision of the condylar surface (Toller and Wilcox, 1978).

In the latter group, when gross erosions were present, specimens were selected from the fibrous surfaces close to the principal articular lesions. In cases with evidence only of early disease, specimens were taken from the slightly fibrillated surfaces in the regions of articular contact.

In general the ultramicroscopic appearances of the tissues taken from those patients with only pain and dysfunction are indistinguishable from material obtained from patients with frank degenerative disease of the temporomandibular joint. The observations may be described in terms of changes in the fibrous stroma and in cellular morphology.

Changes in the Fibrous Stroma

There is a loss of the lamina splendens at the extreme surface and alterations in both the collagen and the ground substance as they are exposed directly to the articular cavity (*Fig. 5.7a*). The collagen fibrils, normally arranged in orderly interlacing bundles, become disrupted and of smaller diameter. They appear to lose their cohesion and are gradually replaced by an electron dense amorphous material (*Fig. 5.7b*).

Changes in Cellular Morphology

Many of the fibroblasts appear normal but others, although their nuclei and plasma membranes remain unchanged, have abnormal cytoplasm. The mitochrondria are swollen and distended with distorted cristae. The rough endoplasmic reticulum contains dilated and irregular cisternae and is frequently found in isolated patches instead of being evenly distributed throughout the cytoplasm.

Other cytoplasmic inclusions have a bubbly appearance (*Fig. 5.7c*). The more superficial cells show greatly increased numbers of vacuoles in their cytoplasm which seem to presage their disintegration at the articular surface. Closely associated with but quite distinct from the abnormal cells in these sections, are vermiform bodies.

Vermiform Bodies

These are serpiginous structures of about 1 μm in diameter and usually found in the deeper layers of the surface. Owing to their configuration,

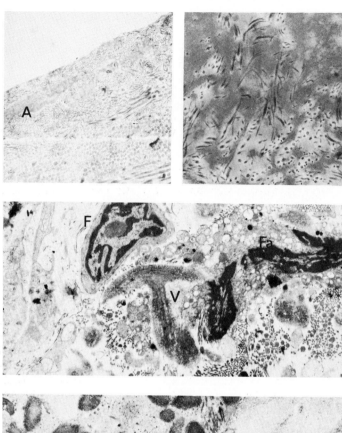

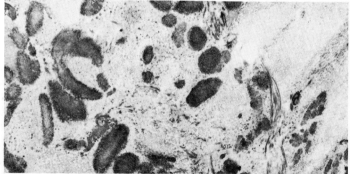

Fig. 5.7. Electron micrographs of articular surface tissue from patients with severe temporomandibular joint pain and dysfunction. *a,* Early changes. Loss of the lamina splendens and replacement of the collagen by amorphous material (**A**). × 7200. *b,* The destruction of the normal orderly interlacing arrangement of collagen fibrils and their replacement with a heavy accumulation of amorphous material. × 14400. *c,* Abnormal fibrocyte (**Fa**) with bubbly cytoplasmic inclusions, adjacent to a branched vermiform body (**V**). Normal fibrocyte (**F**). × 12600. *d,* Oblique sections of vermiform bodies. × 12600.

only small portions are shown on section, some horizontal, some oblique and others transverse (*Fig.* 5.7*d*). Generally they exhibit a fine longitudinal striation and, under light microscopy, and utilizing a suitable stain, it has been possible to demonstrate that they are of an elastic-like nature.

Vermiform bodies differ from the elastic fibres normally found in condylar surfaces and it is suggested that they are formed in response to abnormal stress. Their accumulation seems to create zones of weakness in the fibrous condylar surface which may facilitate its break-up (fibrillation).

Conclusions

The overall ultramicroscopic picture may reasonably be related to the complex biochemical changes that have been observed in the study of osteoarthrosis of other joints. The physical alteration of the ground substance which allows the splitting of the collagen, possibly facilitates the loss of water and proteoglycans from the joint surface. The cells with abnormally arranged and excessive endoplasmic reticulum may be displaying a bizarre hyperactivity in an attempt to compensate for this protein loss.

The important factor, however, is the change in the physical nature of the surface. It has been stated (p. 18) that the frictional properties of the joint are dependent, not only upon the lubricating medium, but the characteristics of the articulating surfaces. The ultramicroscopically altered surfaces are extremely likely to exhibit marked changes to their normal low frictional qualities. It is, therefore, not difficult to visualize intermittent or prolonged sticking between two such surfaces in sliding contact, especially under conditions of excessive muscular loading.

ELECTROMYOGRAPHY

Electromyography is of limited value in the diagnosis of temporo-mandibular joint disorders. Palpation of the temporalis and masseter will give as much information as is needed about the condition of each muscle. The extent and timing of the contractions thus may be compared, one side with the other. As a research tool, however, electromyography has proved to be of value in the investigation of the function of the two separate heads of lateral pterygoid. *Fig.* 5.8*a* shows that the inferior head serves principally to assist jaw opening and, in the normal patient, is relatively inactive in other jaw movements. In those patients with a dysfunction, the inferior head, on the affected side, contracts on closing (*Fig.* 5.8*b*).

The meniscus may be regarded as a modified tendon of insertion of the superior head of lateral pterygoid. Normally, this muscle contracts to stabilize the condyle against the eminence when the teeth

75

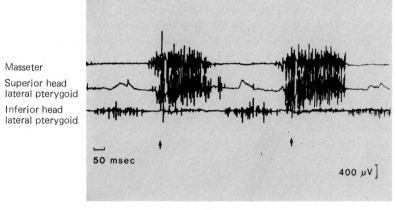

Masseter

Superior head
lateral pterygoid

Inferior head
lateral pterygoid

50 msec

400 µV]

a

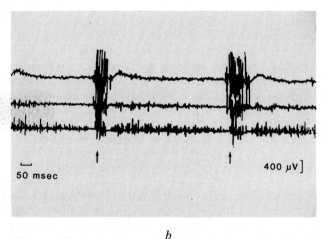

50 msec

400 µV]

b

Fig. 5.8. Electromyographs illustrating the close-clench cycle (*upper trace,* masseter; *middle trace,* superior head of lateral pterygoid; *lower trace,* inferior head of lateral pterygoid). *a,* The normal patient, where the inferior head of the lateral pterygoid contracts anatagonistically to masseter and the superior head. *b,* The patient with a dysfunction, where the inferior head is hyperactive and contracts with the other two muscles as the teeth occlude (*arrowed*). (Reproduced by permission of *Br. J. Oral Maxillofac. Surg.*)

approximate. In the abnormal joint, where the attachments of the meniscus are weakened or lost, the inferior head appears to be recruited to assist in stabilizing the condyle (Juniper, 1984).

The investigation of lateral pterygoid function in this manner is achieved only with fine wire electrodes inserted directly into individual muscles. It is therefore unsuited to clinical practice. Placing surface electrodes over the accessible temporalis and masseter may be of value in using electromyography as biofeedback. Here, the electrical wave forms are transposed into auditory signals and the magnitude of the contraction is gauged by the volume of noise generated. Some clinicians use this method to bring the undesirable hyperactivity of the masticatory muscles to the attention of the patient who then may be able to control the abnormal function.

AN EXPLANATION

Utilizing the information obtained from the preceding special investigations, and clinical and radiographic findings it is possible now to propose an hypothesis that accounts for the features of mandibular stress syndrome. This is illustrated in *Fig.* 5.9.

1. *Meniscal Hesitation*

Repetitive overload on the joint alters the physical nature of the sliding articular surfaces and hence changes their frictional characteristics. This results in meniscal hesitation. The disc becomes liable to stick during its normal range of movement; the joint begins to dysfunction.

The first sign and symptoms is a simple click. There is no associated discomfort and little or no deviation of the jaw. In the initial opening movement, the meniscus, instead of remaining stationary, adheres to the condyle as it rotates (*Fig.* 5.10). As forward translation in the upper compartment begins, a tension builds up in the meniscus and, on further opening, the friction between it and the condyle is overcome with a release of energy. The meniscus clicks backwards suddenly, its thickened posterior band squeezing between the condyle and eminence to assume its normal position as function proceeds. This is the click that is abolished by raising the bite (as described on p. 37). Opening the jaw in the retruded position has a similar effect but in this case there is little or no forward translation in the upper compartment and hence no click.

2. *Damage to the Meniscal Attachments*

A simple click may be followed quickly by other manifestations of mandibular stress syndrome. On the other hand, it may persist for many years without changing substantially. However, either through

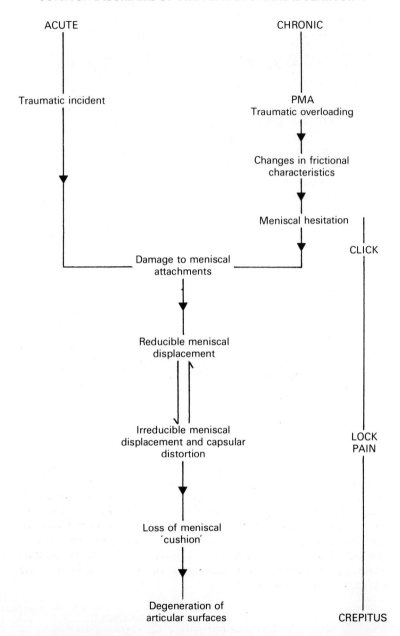

Fig. 5.9. The aetiology and progress of mandibular stress syndrome.

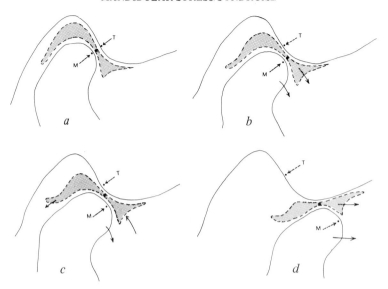

Fig. 5.10. Diagrams illustrating the early click. T is a fixed point on the temporal bone and M on the condylar surface. *a,* Jaw closed position. *b,* In the initial opening movement, which is mainly rotation of the condyle, the meniscus sticks in the lower compartment (i.e. at point M). As forward translation in the upper compartment begins, a tension builds up in the meniscus. *c,* On further opening, the tension is suddenly released with a click as the meniscus snaps backwards to assume its correct relationship with the condyle. *d,* Opening then proceeds as normal.

an acute traumatic incident, or by the persistent chronic trauma of overload and hesitation, the meniscal attachments are damaged. The bilaminar posterior ligament becomes stretched or, more rarely, even torn. Its superior lamella loses its elasticity while the attachment of the inferior lamella to the posterior aspect of the condyle is weakened. This allows the meniscus to displace anteriorly and reciprocal or multiple clicks may be heard as it slips in and out of its normal functional relationship with the articulating surfaces. Eventually the meniscal attachments at the medial and lateral poles of the condyle become weakened and stretched and further displacement is facilitated. The symptoms of stiffness and pain appear.

3. *Reducible Meniscal Displacement*

The meniscus, at rest, now occupies a position anteromedial to the condyle. In the early stages of this anterior displacement, the patient, by manoeuvring the jaw away from and then back to the affected side, is able to reduce the meniscus. It clicks back to assume its normal relationship allowing normal opening to proceed (*Fig.* 5.11*b*). There may be some discomfort as the nociceptive receptors in the distorted capsular tissues are irritated.

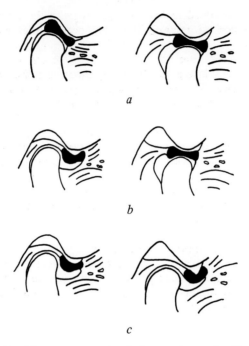

Fig. 5.11. Diagrams extrapolated from arthrographs illustrating the position of the meniscus in relation to the bony articulating surfaces with the jaw closed and open. *a*, The normal joint. *b*, Reducible meniscal displacement. *c*, Irreducible meniscal displacement.

This situation may persist for some time. However, there may be periods when reduction becomes difficult and it takes longer for the meniscus to return to its normal position. The jaw locks.

4. *Irreducible Meniscal Displacement*

With further weakening of all its attachments, the meniscus becomes irreversibly displaced (*Fig.* 5.11*c*). It remains trapped in the antero-medial position. There is little or no forward translation of the condyle, only the initial rotation. The jaw, therefore, opens only a small amount and deviates towards the affected side. There is frequently severe pain as the capsular tissues are distorted and the condyle impinges on the bilaminar ligament with its rich supply of sensory nerve endings. There may be discomfort in the associated muscles due to reflex spasm.

5. *Resolution*

Relief of the overload during the early stages of the syndrome allows normal function to resume. This may occur either spontaneously or following successful treatment. Resolution may even take place following some damage to the meniscal ligaments; in this case, by subarticular remodelling of the joint, modifying the shape of the condylar surface. The more damage the posterior ligament sustains, however, the less likely the problem is to resolve.

6. *Degeneration*

Once the meniscus has become displaced permanently its 'cushioning' function is lost. The loads on the joint then exceed easily the physiological tolerence of the articular surfaces, and degenerative changes take place. This is frequently a self-limiting process and resolves with the formation of a new articular surface, often with gross modification of the overall shape of the condyle.

The preceding description is perhaps an over-simplified account of the process and is somewhat hypothetical. However, it does take into account much recent research and allows the authors to establish a rational approach to the treatment of the common disorders of the temporomandibular joint.

CHAPTER 6

THE TREATMENT

Although a diagnosis of mandibular stress syndrome is not difficult to establish, successful management of most cases is dependent upon a thorough assessment of all the clinical and aetiological findings. It is clear from the hypotheses presented in the previous chapter that a rational approach should be directed towards removal of the overload on the joint, principally by reducing abnormal excessive muscular action. With these points in mind, management may be instigated along the following lines:

1. Treatment of the symptoms.
2. Treatment of the underlying cause.
3. Treatment of the predisposing factors.
4. Treatment of the pathological effects (Chapter 7).

These are only a guide as there are some treatment techniques that overlap more than one of the divisions. There is also no need to proceed in this order. The management of any case must be planned according to the requirements of the particular patient and this is discussed in more detail in the last section of this chapter.

Time and facilities require consideration. A busy consultant clinic in an oral surgery unit is no place to treat a patient with a temporomandibular joint problem. Nor is the crowded atmosphere of most teaching hospital departments. If treatment is carried out in a hospital, then a special clinic should be set aside for the purpose; but perhaps the private surgery (office) is the most suitable environment.

TREATMENT OF THE SYMPTOMS

Generally it is discomfort that motivates a patient to seek treatment. Speedy and efficient management of this aspect not only relieves suffering but also helps gain the patient's confidence. This places the clinician in a more favourable position to assess the underlying problem.

Reassurance

Reassurance is the one line of treatment common to all cases. Frequently the patient is concerned that the condition is serious and reassurance to the contrary does a great deal to diminish anxiety which in itself may be a significant aetiological factor. A simple explanation of the problem is mandatory and must be expressed in terms that the patient can easily understand. A reasonable approach, for example, is to describe it as a disorder caused by putting too much strain on the joint. The object of treatment is to find out why this is happening and to remove the causes.

It is advisable, at this early stage, to avoid expressions such as anxiety and depression since these may indicate to the patient that the clinician does not feel that the symptoms are 'real'. The problem of explaining the psychic aspects of the condition will be described later.

Prognosis may also be discussed. It should be pointed out that it is a very common disorder which usually responds well to treatment. However, there are no magic cures and several visits at least will be necessary to get the problem under control.

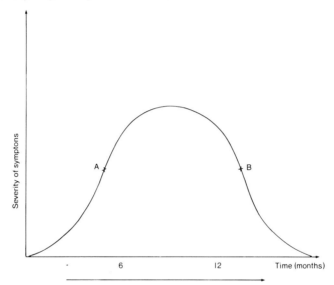

Fig. 6.1. Graph used in explaining the prognosis of degenerative change in the temporomandibular joint to the patient (*see text* for explanation).

If degenerative change is diagnosed then it should be explained that the symptoms may get worse before improving although in all cases the joint eventually heals. A useful way of illustrating this is to draw a graph (*Fig.* 6.1). It is conceded that at the present time it is difficult to assess the patient's exact position. If at point A, the condition will deteriorate before it improves; but if at point B, it is well on the way to getting better. It must be stressed, however, that with the proper management, progress is always in the same direction, from left to right.

Resting the Jaw

The first appointment is usually concerned only with diagnosis and reassurance but these may be augmented with advice to rest the jaw and simple medication. Resting, in this context, implies avoiding excessive jaw movements such as yawning, or those required to chew hard foods. Indeed, these may already be painful and the patient can thus be advised to refrain from any activity that hurts. A soft diet is recommended and all foods cut into small pieces. An apple should be sliced and not bitten whole. If possible, all jaw movements that cause clicking should be avoided, although this may be difficult. It might even be suggested that the patient refrain from shouting at the spouse and children, but this may be more difficult still. A useful analogy in explaining the regime to the patient is the sprained ankle. This gets better much more quickly if it is rested by putting one's feet up, rather than by continuing to walk on it.

Medication

The use of simple anodynes such as aspirin and paracetamol to control pain is recommended, as necessary. More useful may be the prescription of a sedative such as diazepam 5 mg to be taken nightly for two weeks in the first instance. This regime often relieves early morning jaw stiffness when there is a nocturnal bruxing habit, probably by a combination of its muscle relaxing and tranquillizing effects. It is wise to suggest that any such drug is taken at the latest possible moment before retiring so as not to interfere with normal behaviour (in particular, sex life) which in itself may increase anxiety to the overall detriment of treatment. A hypnotic (e.g. nitrazepam) may help where insomnia or restlessness is a problem.

Where degenerative joint change is present, more powerful analgesia may be necessary. Occasionally specific antiarthritic preparations are helpful. A common example is indomethacin (Indocid; Indocin) 25–50 mg thrice daily with meals.

At the second visit, 2–4 weeks later, the condition is assessed for improvement. If this is found then the patient is congratulated. Much can be achieved by encouraging a person in this manner and leading him on with a positive approach. More active treatment should now be considered.

Remedial Exercises

The rationale behind remedial exercise is to promote normal mandibular function. It may also help the patient to relax the jaw muscles. The following approach is only one of many that have been advocated.

    a. The patient is first instructed to relax the mandibular muscles. He is asked to clench his teeth while palpating the masseters and then the temporales. These are felt to 'harden' and then 'soften' on relaxation (*Fig.* 6.2).

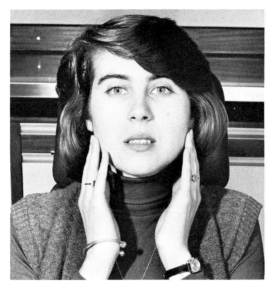

Fig. 6.2. Learning to relax the mandibular muscles by feeling them 'harden' and 'soften'.

b. From the relaxed position the patient is instructed to open the mouth without deviating the chin. A vertical line drawn over the lips with an indelible pencil or lipstick helps to accentuate the movements (*Fig.* 6.3*a*). Care must be taken not to protrude the mandible. It is stressed that the amount of opening is unimportant but if there is deviation to one side or the other (*Fig.* 6.3*b*) then this should not be corrected but the exercise must be started again from the relaxed position.

c. The advice is to spend five to ten minutes a day doing this exercise in quiet surroundings, in front of a dressing table mirror. The procedure is not usually as easy to perform as it sounds, and attempts to achieve a straight up and down opening may initially be quite frustrating. Perseverence is therefore required.

Heat Treatment

Heat treatment may be successful in relieving pain and stiffness in the muscles. The most frequently used method is short-wave diathermy but ultrasonics seem to have a similar effect. Probably just as helpful is self-massage of the affected area (usually over the masseter) using a small amount of cream containing a counter irritant such as methyl salicylate. This is a positive measure, easily carried out by the patient. The value of the more sophisticated techniques may be partly psychological in that the patient is made to feel that more is being done.

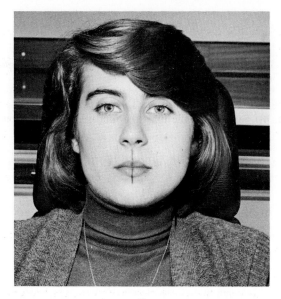

a

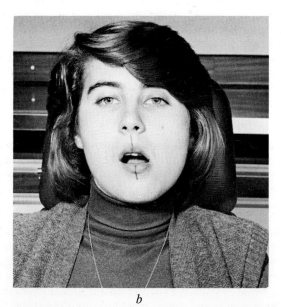

b

Fig. 6.3. *a,* A vertical line drawn over the lips as an aid to exercising the jaw in the vertical plane. *b,* Deviation of the mandible to the left.

The Occlusal Splint or Bite Plane

There can be little doubt that the occlusal splint or bite plane is one of the most useful methods for treating temporomandibular joint disorders. Several different designs have been suggested and Greene (1973) has demonstrated some interesting results in a study of three types. The first group of patients were treated with a splint that covered only the soft tissues of the palate. Although this had no direct effect on the occlusion, 40 per cent of the patients improved. In the second group, who were treated with an appliance that covered only the anterior teeth and which discluded the posteriors, there was a positive response in 50 per cent of the patients. The positive response in the third group, which were treated with a splint providing full occlusal coverage, was 80 per cent.

Although these observations suggested that a placebo effect may be achieved with the use of an appliance, the physical effects of a splint constructed to influence the occlusion in a controlled manner is more likely to provide successful treatment.

In the past, perhaps the most popular splint was that constructed to cover the occlusal surfaces of all the maxillary teeth, and it was obviously important that the thickness of the occlusal coverage was less than that of the freeway space. The splint was designed on articulated models to allow free lateral sliding and protrusive movements of the cusps of the lower teeth against the acrylic of the occlusal plane. It proved to be a very useful appliance but was rather clumsy and thus frequently poorly tolerated by the patient.

It was noted by some clinicians that a deliberate easing of this bite plane over the posterior teeth at subsequent visits tended to speed resolution of the symptoms, and this observation led to the recommendation that the most useful and best tolerated appliance is the upper anterior bite plane which occludes only on the lower six anterior teeth. All the posterior teeth are discluded and the palatal acrylic may be cut clear of the cervical aspects of the premolars to reduce bulk. It is best retained by Adams' cribs on the upper first molars (*Fig. 6.4*). When fitted, the anterior bite plane is ground in with the aid of articulating paper so as to provide an even contact with the lower anterior teeth.

It is also the present authors' view that this type of appliance is the most satisfactory of all the designs although its use is generally limited to night time and short periods during the day. Should a patient require an appliance for daytime use, then a simple total occlusal splint (*Fig. 6.5*) either of soft or hard vinyl plastic, made on a vacuum-forming machine, is often well tolerated. This splint, which may be worn either over upper or lower teeth, may be refined by adding autopolymerizing resin to its occlusal surface and functionally generating indentations in the resin while it is setting.

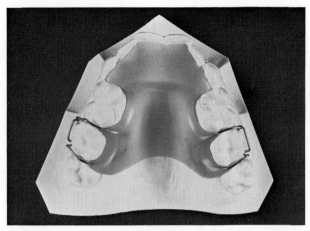

Fig. 6.4. The upper anterior bite plane.

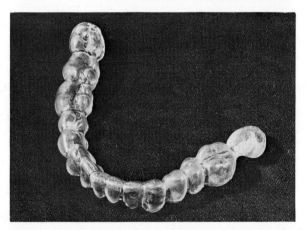

Fig. 6.5. A vacuum-formed total occlusal splint constructed of soft vinyl plastic.

Whichever type of splint is selected, however, regular adjustments of the bite and clasps during the first few weeks of use may be necessary if the maximum benefit is to be gained. Once the symptoms of dysfunction begin to disappear, the mandible frequently assumes a new position which must be catered for at the occlusal contact level.

The indications for using a bite plane are as follows:

   a. Treating a click. Raising the bite frequently abolishes an early click. The use of a splint at night and as much as possible during the day will often relieve this symptom.

b. Prevention of bruxing. Many dysfunctions present with symptoms which are worse on waking and thus suggest a nocturnal bruxing habit. The majority of these cases may be treated successfully with the use of a bite plane at night only. It may be valuable to prescribe diazepam or nitrazepam, 5 mg *nocte,* for 4 or 5 days when the appliance is first fitted. This regime helps the patient to overcome the initial difficulties of sleeping with a strange object in the mouth.

c. The relief of pain. Occasionally, if other conservative methods fail, a bite appliance may give symptomatic relief.

The bite plane probably inhibits the simple early click by preventing full backward rotation of the condyle within the articular fossa. How it acts to relieve other symptoms is not clear although a number of conjectures are possible. At a subconscious level, during sleep, it may draw attention to abnormal clenching or grinding habits which are consequently modified or cease entirely. It may, by discluding all but the anterior teeth, neutralize or reduce noxious sensory inputs and thereby interrupt the normal neuromuscular reflex mechanism.

A more logical and simpler approach suggests that the appliance acts by two mechanisms:

1. By relieving the load on the joint.
2. By helping to maintain the normal meniscal-condylar relationship.

In the case of a nocturnal bruxing habit, for example, the articular surfaces of the joint are so affected by the repetitive nature of the overload that their normal free-sliding properties are impaired. Muscle fatigue and reflex spasm add to the problem. The bite plane acts mechanically to relieve the joint of much of this load. It prevents direct trauma to the fibrous structure of the surfaces thus allowing normal movement.

At an early stage of internal derangement the meniscus, which is displaced anteriorly at the beginning of the opening cycle, clicks back into the normal meniscal-condylar relationship as forward translation proceeds. The bite plane, when correctly designed, prevents the initial meniscal displacement. Continued wearing of the appliance may allow the damaged posterior attachment to stabilize and bony remodelling to take place thus resolving the disorder.

Manzione et al. (1984c) have described a method for registering the optimal mandibular position for the ideal meniscal-condylar relationship. The correct occlusal relationship, to which the bite splint is constructed, is assessed utilizing an arthrographic technique.

Whatever the precise mode of action, there is little doubt that the occlusal splint is a valuable means of treatment. Its prolonged use, however, may lead to damage of the teeth and supporting structures and it is important to wean the patient off the appliance as early as possible.

TREATMENT OF THE UNDERLYING CAUSE

The neuromuscular activity, which leads to the repetitive overloading of the joint, is primarily induced by emotional stress and tension. Relief of these factors must therefore be the principal aim when treating the underlying cause of the syndrome. Since the average clinician who treats temporomandibular joint disorders is likely to have had little formal psychiatric training, this is probably the most difficult phase in the management of the problem.

The stresses and tensions to which any individual is subjected may, for the purpose of this description, be divided into two groups. There are those related to everyday situations and those due to exceptional circumstances. Everyday stresses affect all people at all times although tolerance and response vary widely. Examples are personal relationships, financial difficulties, occupational problems and examinations. The list is endless and indeed the tensions that they create are all part of normal life. The problem may have reached a peak in our 'Western culture' and this is possibly why mandibular stress syndrome is so prevalent in these countries.

The second group are the emotional stresses brought on by exceptional circumstances such as a family bereavement, a severe illness or a sudden change in individual fortune. The onset of a temporomandibular joint disorder is frequently coincident with one of these situations.

The individuals with which we are dealing possess a specific physiological response to these anxieties. Making them aware of this and showing genuine concern for their problem may be the most important aspect of the treatment.

Explaining the Psychic Aspect of the Disorder

This phase of treatment is best handled when the symptoms are under control and the patient is gaining confidence in the clinician. It must be dealt with in a very careful and sympathetic manner since any suggestion that the disorder might be psychological is likely to arouse resentment or even hostility in a large proportion of patients. The reaction of these people is to believe that the clinician suspects their symptoms to be imaginary and frequent reassurance to the contrary is essential.

Every clinician will develop an individual approach but the following technique is that used by one of the authors (HDO). It is only a guide and must be varied from one patient to another according to individual circumstances, situations and intelligence.

'All of us are subject to various mental stresses and strains every day of our lives. We have to cope with them all, jobs, families, money, mortgages and personal problems, just to name a few. You are no different in this respect to me or anyone else.

'The tensions that these stresses and strains create have to have an outlet and the way they manifest themselves in you is through overactivity of your jaw muscles, even when you are relaxing or sleeping. This overactivity puts an increased strain on the joint which begins to function abnormally and produces the symptoms from which you have been suffering.

'I think it unlikely that you have more serious problems than most other people, it is just that you respond to these everyday stresses and strains in this particular way. Other people may smoke a lot, drink or respond in different ways. You have this habit in certain situations of contracting your jaw muscles and clenching your teeth'.

Having been given this explanation, the patient is asked to think over what has been said and, if possible, discuss it with the spouse before the next appointment. In other words, individuals are requested to investigate their own problem, to find out in what situations they clench their teeth or perform other irrelevent jaw movements. It is surprising how many of them confirm the clinician's suspicions at the next visit and how successful this technique is as a therapy itself.

MEDICAL MANAGEMENT

The symptoms of the majority of patients improve with a combination of the above explanation and the physical therapy described in the first section of this chapter. However, if after several visits there is little or no improvement, then a medical management utilizing anti-depressant drugs should be considered. Criteria for this approach have been described by Harris (1985). He stresses the necessity to:

1. Identify not only the features of the facial (TMJ) pain but also chronic pain disorders elsewhere, for example, the head, neck, back, spastic colon and the pelvis;
2. Identify predisposing adverse life events and any history of emotional or psychiatric disturbance;
3. Emphasize to the patient that the pain is real, not imaginary, arising in 'cramped' muscle and dilated blood vessels as a response to emotional stress;
4. Emphasize that the drug therapy is not being used to treat depression but has a direct effect in relieving the painful muscles and blood vessels.

The tricyclic antidepressants or, alternatively, monoamine oxidase inhibitors (MAOIs) may be used, although there seems to be no clear indication as to why one group is preferable to the other in the management of a particular case. With a suitable interval, both may be tried but care should be taken with their use as there are several complications and contraindications. Their prescription is best confined to those clinicians experienced in their effects.

If a severe depressive disorder or other psychosis is suspected, the patient should be referred urgently to a psychiatrist.

HYPNOTHERAPY

Hypnosis is a state of altered consciousness that may be induced, in susceptible patients, by a variety of techniques. These include relaxation, slow deep respiration, a fixation point for attention and rhythmic monotonous instruction with a graded series of suggestions. In the hands of suitably trained and skilled clinicians, hypnosis may be employed for psychotherapeutic purposes. For example, post-hypnotic suggestion is used frequently to treat behavioural problems such as smoking, drinking and over-eating.

Bruxism, the underlying cause of a large proportion of temporomandibular joint disorders, is a response to the various emotional and stressful situations that are met with in everyday life. Grinding the teeth may be an introverted form of aggression engendered by these problems.

The patient first must be made aware of the problems and how these have become manifested in bruxism. One technique then is to place the subject into a light or medium trance and to suggest that, instead of grinding the teeth, the fist is clenched. Self-hypnosis may be taught so that at night the patient will awaken if bruxing commences. This will not occur if, as suggested, the fist is clenched. Several of the author's patients have responded successfully to this treatment and it is probable that a significant proportion of temporomandibular joint problems would benefit from a similar approach. Further investigation and trial are necessary.

TREATMENT OF THE PREDISPOSING FACTORS

The underlying cause of mandibular stress syndrome, the stress-induced neuromuscular overload, may be influenced by various predisposing factors. These may create situations which render an individual more prone to the disorder but may also precipitate or prolong its effects.

The principal predisposing factor is the occlusion, modification of which has been practised widely in the management of temporomandibular joint conditions. Treatments have ranged from simple equilibration to full-mouth reconstruction, alteration of the vertical dimension, orthodontics or a combination of these procedures (Goodman et al., 1976). Occlusal therapy in this context, however, is a controversial subject, especially since it has been difficult to produce clinical evidence to show that it is of any value. Indeed, the findings of the same authors suggest that it might have nothing more than a placebo effect.

The clinical impression of the present authors, on the other hand, is that certain occlusal procedures are useful and often necessary in the total treatment of a temporomandibular joint problem. Efforts should be made to restore and maintain adequate and satisfactory function, especially where degenerative change has occurred. Generally, except where extractions are indicated, only reversible procedures should be carried out. It is rarely necessary, in the treatment of mandibular stress syndrome itself, to recommend, often at considerable financial cost, prolonged oral rehabilitation and occlusal equilibration programmes which demand irreversible techniques.

Caries and other Oral Pathology

All dental decay must be eliminated and suspect or unsatisfactory restorations replaced. Grossly infected teeth should be removed and any other dental or oral pathology dealt with. These factors are all potential sources of discomfort and may affect the way in which a patient bites or chews. Especially relevant are third molars with histories of pericoronitis. It should be noted, however, that mandibular stress syndrome may be exacerbated by prolonged courses of dental treatment and so the length of each session should be kept to a minimum.

Displaced teeth, such as an overerupted and unopposed molar, may cause similar problems and should be removed. The same applies to buccally displaced upper third molars which may tend to traumatize the inside of the cheek.

Prostheses

Prosthetic restoration or replacement is necessary should it be judged that the number and site of the missing teeth or the present appliance is detrimental to function. This is generally so in cases where there is a lack of posterior occlusal support or the patient is wearing worn, ill-designed or poorly fitting dentures. Overclosures may create the situation that predisposes the joint to a far greater load than is usual. A loose prosthesis may induce parafunctional muscle activity or abnormal function in efforts to stabilize it during mastication or even at rest. An overlay prosthesis might be considered where there is gross dental attrition.

Occlusal Adjustment

Occlusal adjustment is rarely necessary. High restorations will have generally manifested themselves well before a temporomandibular joint disorder develops but may conceivably initiate or exacerbate the problem. It is difficult otherwise, to visualize how significant occlusal interference might develop in a previously functional dentition unless iatrogenically produced. Adjustment of an obvious prematurity does occasionally provide relief but should only be undertaken after careful diagnosis and planning. Much damage has been done by indiscriminate grinding of tooth surface.

Other Predisposing Factors

Other factors that may play a part in exacerbating the problem are the occupational and recreational pastimes discussed in Chapter 3. Most of these may simply be avoided but it may be necessary to refrain, either temporarily or permanently from hobbies such as playing a wind instrument or opera singing. The authors have both treated a number of chronic gum chewers by recommending they find another outlet for their aggressions.

TREATMENT PLANNING

The preceding sections of the chapter will have revealed the wide variety of techniques that are available for the management of a temporomandibular joint disorder. In order that these may be utilized to their best advantage, it is as well to develop a treatment plan according to a set pattern. For descriptive purposes, management may be divided into three phases:

1. Examination and diagnosis.
2. Active treatment.
3. Resolution.

These are not rigid divisions since there is often an overlap between one phase and the next. There are also frequent cases that respond so well to the simple measures of Phase 1 that no active treatment is required. Only experience, however, will tell the clinician which treatments within each phase are appropriate for a particular patient.

PHASE 1. EXAMINATION AND DIAGNOSIS

a. Explanation and reassurance.
b. Simple measures for the relief of symptoms.

During these first visits while assessing the clinical findings and aetiological factors, an explanation of the problem and reassurance should allay anxiety and help in gaining a patient's confidence. This is frequently augmented with simple measures to relieve symptoms, such as instruction to rest the jaw and medication in the form of minor analgesics, tranquillizers and hypnotics.

PHASE 2. ACTIVE TREATMENT

a. Management of the predisposing factors.
b. Bite appliances.
c. Remedial exercises.

d. Explanation of the psychic aspect.

e. Psychotropic medication.

Before continuing with active treatment of the symptoms and underlying cause, it is usually best to deal with any predisposing factor. This is most frequently concerned with the provision or maintenance of an adequate functional occlusion. For example, it is the stage of the treatment where partially erupted third molars are removed or, if necessary an inadequate prosthesis is replaced.

In the absence of any improvement, perseverence with a bite appliance should not be continued for more than 3–4 weeks. Occasionally it is worth constructing an alternative design as some patients tolerate one type better than another.

The aspect of therapy that is mandatory in all cases is an explanation of the psychic nature of the problem. It is repeated to the patient on several occasions if necessary, with discussion as to how the habitual muscular activity might be controlled. The response to this form of treatment seems to be directly related to how well the patient understands, or wants to understand the problem.

Psychotropic medication may be indicated if an underlying anxiety or depressive state is suspected. This often only becomes apparent after several visits, when there has been little progress. Consultation, at this stage, with the patient's medical practitioner is frequently helpful.

PHASE 3. RESOLUTION

a. Weaning from appliances and drugs.

b. Supportive therapy.

c. Reassurance as to prognosis.

This phase is reached when the symptoms have subsided and, just as importantly, the patient understands the problem. Medication, if prescribed, is gradually withdrawn. Attempts are then made to leave out the bite appliance, usually on an every-other-night basis. Finally it may be dispensed with altogether.

Where degenerative change has occurred, a different situation exists. In the majority of such cases, symptoms are controlled conservatively, over a longer period, that is until the joint heals. During this time the patient may well require constant encouragement and reassurance (supportive therapy) as to the eventual outcome.

Finally, when the condition has been successfully treated, the problem of recurrence should be discussed. The patient is warned that the predisposition to the disorder will remain. Their response to stress by increased activity of the mandibular musculature may persist. Hopefully, however, a means of correcting the situation has been established and a prolonged course of treatment will not be required a second time.

CHAPTER 7

THE TREATMENT OF THE PATHOLOGICAL EFFECTS

Not all cases of mandibular stress syndrome respond to the conservative therapies described in the previous chapter. A certain proportion continue to suffer the symptoms to a greater or lesser degree and indeed there are those patients in whom intractable pain becomes quite intolerable. Often a deep-seated psychiatric condition is the real problem and it is worthwhile referring these cases to a psychiatrist or another clinician with a greater experience in this branch of medicine.

It is difficult to assess the number of patients who do not respond well since they are liable to pass from one doctor to another seeking treatment. The general impression is that the figure is between 5 and 10 per cent although by no means do they all follow on to non-conservative management. Studies have been made to assess the success rate of conservative therapy, examples are reports by Thomson (1971) and Zarb and Thompson (1975). In the former, 7 out of 100 patients failed to respond and in the latter study 10 out of 93. Zarb and Thompson also carried out a longitudinal follow-up (24—84 months) in which 26 of the original 93 patients had a frank recurrence which led them to seek therapy prior to their recall appointments. Clinical and/or radiographical evidence of degenerative change in the condylar surface is frequently discovered in this residual group of patients. Just as often, on the other hand, there are no such helpful findings although degeneration cannot be ruled out. A number of surgical procedures have been devised to treat these situations but at this stage it is worth considering a corticosteroid injection into the affected joint.

INTRA-ARTICULAR CORTICOSTEROID

In 1951, Hollander and his associates described the effects of intra-articular injections of cortisone and hydrocortisone in rheumatoid joints. The latter drug proved to be the far more effective of the two in relieving local signs and symptoms of inflammation. Pharmacological studies revealed that the local tissues were not able to convert cortisone acetate to the natural cortisol and hence the greater efficacy of hydrocortisone.

The injection of a corticosteroid into the temporomandibular joint was first reported by Horton (1953). Since then, a number of papers have related varying degrees of success with the use of hydrocortisone and its related synthetic steroid compounds, prednisolone, triamcinolone and betamethasone.

Poswillo (1970) expressed concern that in spite of the clinical success of the technique, there was evidence that alterations in the size and shape of the mandibular condyle had taken place, even though the patients had remained symptom free for long periods. His research into the effects of intra-articular steroids in a near-human primate, the *Macaca irus* monkey, demonstrated that multiple injections are followed by gross circumferential destruction of the condylar articular cap of fibrocartilage. This is superseded by repair, which restores the normal arrangement of the condylar head, but on a smaller scale than the original.

Results of other studies by Salter et al. (1967) on rabbits and Gibson et al. (1976) again on the *Macaca irus* monkey, produced findings that were contradictory in respect of the effects of multiple or single injections. It therefore seems likely that there is a significant variation in drug susceptibility among species, such that the possible reference of animal experiments to man must be made with caution. In his report of 160 cases of intra-articular corticosteroid therapy, Toller (1977b) stated that there is no evidence to show that a single injection causes damage that can be detected radiographically to an apparently sound articular surface. It is still possible, however, that multiple injections can cause damage to the temporomandibular joint, and should therefore be avoided.

Technique

1. *Asepsis*

Elective entry into a joint must be performed under strict aseptic conditions. It is recommended that a surgical trolley is laid up as indicated in *Fig. 7.1.*

2. *Local Anaesthesia*

Local anaesthesia of the joint is obtained by an auriculotemporal nerve block. The pre-auricular skin is prepared with a suitable antiseptic solution, such as 1 per cent aqueous Hibitane, and the condyle palpated through the skin during opening, closing and lateral movements of the jaw. A 40 mm needle, fitted to an aspirating cartridge syringe containing 2 per cent lignocaine with 1:8000 adrenaline, is passed through the skin about 4mm in front of the tragus (*Fig. 7.2a*) and directed inwards and forwards until the condyle is felt by the needle tip, a small quantity of anaesthetic solution being injected during this passage. The patient is asked to move the jaw to elicit movement of the condyle against the needle as a check of the position. The needle is then slightly withdrawn and passed behind the head of the condyle for a further penetration of 1 cm where 1 ml of solution is deposited in the region of the auriculo-temporal nerve. Injection near the neck of the condyle instead of behind the lower part of its head produces unwanted diffusion around the facial nerve.

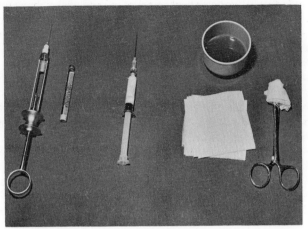

Fig. 7.1. A surgical trolley laid up for the intra-articular injection of corticosteroid.

The effect of the anaesthetic injection is noted. Abolition of pain and increased freedom of jaw movement frequently results, and suggests that reflex muscle spasm is an important factor contributing to the locked jaw. It is wise to reassure the patient that any weakness of the upper facial muscles, or difficulty in closing the eyelid on that side, is a common and transient effect and will disappear within 2–3 hours.

3. *Corticosteroid Injection*
An aqueous suspension of a suitable corticosteroid is drawn up into a syringe fitted with a 40 mm needle of a thick enough gauge (21 g) to allow sensations produced by the instrumentation of fibrous or bony tissue to be easily conveyed to the clinician's fingers. In practice, a disposable syringe system containing an aqueous suspension of methyl-prednisolone acetate is used (Depo-Medrone, 2 ml–40 mg/ml; Depo-Medrol U-Ject. 1 ml–80 mg/ml).

a. LOWER JOINT CAVITY
With the information already obtained from a local anaesthetic injection, that is the exact location of the condylar head, the needle is passed slightly upwards and forwards, with the flat of the bevel towards the bone, until the posterolateral aspect of the condyle is encountered (*Fig.* 7.2*b*). When the bone is felt, the patient is again asked to move the jaw very slightly so that the placing of the needle is confirmed. Then, with small in-and-out movements to avoid catching the periosteum, the tip of the needle is 'walked' upwards and backwards on the condyle until it can be slid over the posterior superior aspect and be in contact

with it. After a further penetration of 5 mm with the needle, the plunger of the syringe is lightly pressed and, if the tip of the needle is in the lower synovial cavity, the fluid will enter freely, without resistance. An injection of 0·5 ml is made at this point.

b. UPPER JOINT CAVITY

A similar injection is made at the same time into the upper joint cavity. For this purpose the needle is partly withdrawn and the patient asked to open the jaw widely. The needle is then directed upwards and forwards towards the anterior part of the roof of the glenoid fossa (*Fig. 7.2c*). The mouth-open position has so advanced the condyle that the needle passes behind the bone without touching it and through the upper part of the capsule behind its attachment to the meniscus which is also in a forward position. The correct point is reached when bone is encountered and the needle is at approximately twice the depth of the

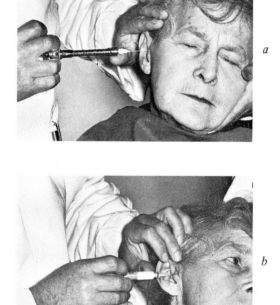

a

b

Fig. 7.2. (see over)

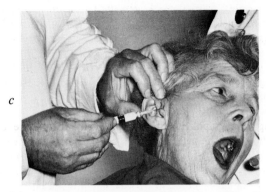

Fig. 7.2. *a,* Local anaesthesia of the joint and overlying tissues. *b,* The injection of corticosteroid into the lower joint cavity. *c,* The injection of corticosteroid into the upper joint cavity.

injection into the lower cavity. If bone is reached before this, then it is possible that the needle has encountered the outer rim of the glenoid cavity. If so, it has to be lowered slightly so it can slide beneath the rim into the fossa where an injection of another 0·5 ml of corticosteroid is deposited. It is frequently necessary to disimpact the needle from the roof of the glenoid fossa to facilitate free injection.

After-effects
There should be little discomfort during the procedure if the local anaesthetic has been effective. The patient, however, may complain of a feeling of pressure from within the joint and will be unable to occlude the teeth properly on the ipsilateral side. This is almost certainly a good sign since it confirms that the injection has been correctly made into the joint capsule.

When the anaesthetic has worn off and for the subsequent 24—48 hours, a great deal of discomfort must be expected and the patient should be warned of this and prescribed a suitable analgesic. Gradually, however, symptoms diminish and if the procedure has been successful, the joint should be pain free, even for a limited period.

A long-term follow-up on 160 patients was reported by Toller (1977b) with the following results:

Age of patient	Good result (cured)	Improved (worthwhile)	Failed
All patients	47%	22%	31%
35 and over	62%	14%	24%
34 and under	21%	32%	47%
40 and over	62%	19%	19%
Under 25	17%	33%	50%

It should be noted from these figures that it is unwise to judge the results in a single group of all ages. Clearly, intra-articular corticosteroid treatment gives poor results in the young compared with the older patient.

In a group of 100 patients, of all ages, who showed an initial satisfactory response to the treatment, 43 complained that painful symptoms had returned after 8–12 weeks whereas in 57, relief was permanent.

Follow-up radiographs taken at subsequent visits were compared with those taken of the articular surface before injection. It was shown that latter development of condylar erosion on a few previously normal surfaces was of the same order as would have been expected in untreated patients with clinical evidence of degenerative disease but with no early radiographic change.

Summary

Summarizing the results, it has been shown that in certain cases, where there is intractable pain, a single intra-articular injection of a suitable corticosteroid into the temporomandibular joint may provide permanent relief. The treatment is most successful in patients over 30 years of age; the older the patient, the greater likelihood of clinical improvement. The technique is not recommended in younger age groups.

The technique is not easy to master unless practised frequently and it is likely that extracapsular injections are often inadvertently made. Perhaps this is the reason why the treatment has gained a poor reputation with so many clinicians.

Where there is radiographic evidence of an erosion before the injection, an advance in the lesion with a reduction in condylar size may be expected but this is consistent with a reduction in symptoms, especially the pain. The final result, after healing has occurred, may indeed resemble a pharmacologically-achieved arthroplasty (*Fig.* 7.3).

TEMPOROMANDIBULAR JOINT SURGERY

Surgery, generally, in mandibular stress syndrome, should be resorted to only when the patient has failed to respond to conservative therapy. It will not resolve the underlying cause of the problem but may relieve and repair its pathological manifestations.

The situation should be discussed at length with the patient and the risks and prognosis of a surgical procedure explained. Many authorities believe an arthrograph, to demonstrate the extent of damage to the joint, to be mandatory at this stage. However, it is the severity of the symptoms and the clinician's inability to provide significant relief by other means that facilitates the decision.

Over the last 40 years, several surgical procedures have passed in

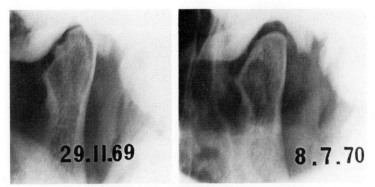

Fig. 7.3. Transpharyngeal radiographs demonstrating the healed condyle of a 58-year-old patient who was treated with an intra-articular corticosteroid injection on 29.11.69.

and out of fashion. These include meniscectomy condylotomy and high condylectomy. Frequently, results have been disappointing and still there is no consensus of opinion as to which is the most useful procedure and for which cases it is most appropriate.

If the reasoned approach taken in this book is adhered to, then an operation on the temporomandibular joint should have the following aims:

1. To remodel the condylar articular surface.
2. To repair the damaged meniscus and/or ligaments.

It is possible that all operations on the temporomandibular joint have the added advantage of sectioning the sensory nerve supply. Not only does this render the joint temporarily free from pain, but also it may interrupt the neuromuscular reflex arc, thereby reducing harmful muscle action.

The Surgical Approach to the Joint

Several surgical approaches to the temporomandibular joint have been devised, including the endaural, the postauricular, the intra-oral and the submandibular. Although they all have their uses, by far the most popular is the preauricular incision. The procedure, which is relatively safe and simple, offers sufficient exposure of the capsule for all the operations that may be used to treat the condition and leaves a scar that is almost totally disguised. Apart from the closed condylotomy technique which is described later in this chapter, only the preauricular approach will be described.

In preparation of the skin, only a minimal amount of hair, consistent with a 'clean' surgical technique, should be removed. Personal appearance, especially for females, has many psychological implications, and since the condition under treatment has a large psychic component, the effect postoperatively of shaving a large portion of the temporal area may aggravate the problem. Long strands of hair may be 'soaped' and retracted beneath a head drape. A sterile pledget of cotton-wool is placed in the external auditory meatus to prevent the ingress of blood.

1. In consultation with the anaesthetist, a 1 : 200 000 solution of adrenaline may be injected subcutaneously to reduce bleeding, and after a pause to allow the drug to act, the incision is made in two parts, B to C and B to A, as illustrated in *Fig.* 7.4. The inferior limit (C) of the incision should carry no further than the lower margin of the tragus.

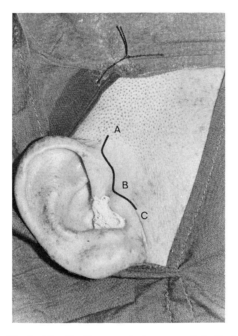

Fig. 7.4. The incision for the preauricular approach to the temporo-mandibular joint (*see text* for description).

Deep extension in the same direction may damage the facial nerve as it turns the posterior border of the parotid. The superior limit (A) curves forward for about 1 cm at the junction of the superior margin of the helix with the skin. Further anterior extension is not usually required for most temporomandibular joint operations but may be made if wider exposure of the capsule and zygomatic arch is necessary.

2. The superior part of the incision is extended through the subcutaneous tissues to the temporalis fascia. Inferiorly the dissection is developed in the plane anterior to the cartilaginous external auditory

canal. The auricular muscle insertions are incised over the root of the zygoma. In this approach the superficial temporal vessels (*see Fig.* 1.8) are retracted anteriorly in the flap but it may be necessary to divide and ligate several small branches. The auriculotemporal nerve is usually not seen but runs vertically, deep to the preauricular muscles.

3. The temporal fascia is then incised, from a point about 2 cm in front of the helix and 1 cm above the zygomatic arch, downwards and backwards to the root of the zygoma. Here, the incision is continued through the periosteum, hard onto bone. A periosteal elevator is then used to lift the periosteum from the zygomatic arch as far as the articular eminence.

4. It is now possible to check the position of the joint by palpation, while manually opening and closing the jaw. With blunt dissection, the superior pole of the parotid and associated soft tissues are reflected anteriorly and inferiorly, thereby exposing the capsule. Further delineation of the capsule, especially posteriorly, is frequently accompanied by a brisk venous haemorrhage. Normally this is controlled easily with pressure.

The capsule now is exposed (*Fig.* 7.5) and according to the chosen procedure, the next stage is carried out.

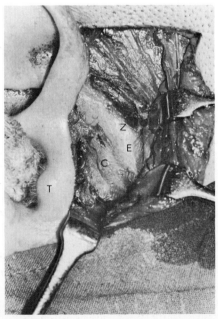

Fig. 7.5 The surgical exposure of the joint capsule. Z, Zygomatic arch; E, Articular eminence; C, Capsule; T, Tragus.

High Condylectomy and Meniscal Repair

The following procedure is appropriate for a case with minimal condylar damage but complete anterior dislocation of the meniscus (*Fig.* 7.6). However, it may be modified according to the findings at operation.

1. The capsule is incised horizontally along the complete length of its lateral aspect just below the edge of its superior attachment. This should leave enough of the capsule superiorly to facilitate suture repair at the end of the procedure. The superior joint compartment is entered and inspected, and the position of the meniscus noted.

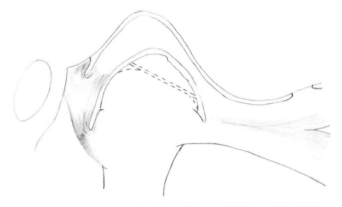

Fig. 7.6. Diagram illustrating the technique of high condylectomy.

2. The lower cut edge of the capsule is retracted inferiorly exposing the lateral attachment of the meniscus. This is incised horizontally down to condylar bone. The meniscus and damaged posterior ligaments are then lifted gently from the articular surface of the condyle which may be inspected for signs of degeneration.

3. A suitable retractor (*Fig.* 7.7a) is passed behind the head of the condyle within the capsule. Not only does this retract and protect the soft tissues but acts as a lever that enables the condyle to be offered firmly against the cutting instrument. It has the added advantage of being a directional guide for manipulating the handpiece (*Fig.* 7.7b).

4. The superior surface of the condyle (as shown in *Fig.* 7.6) is excised using a long shanked, tungsten-carbide tipped, tapered fissure burr. The anatomy of the condyle, especially its mediolateral depth, must be kept in mind, otherwise, by incorrect angulation of the handpiece, it is easy to excise only the lateral portion of the surface (*Fig.* 7.8). The fragment is levered carefully from the capsule, if necessary stripping off remaining muscle attachment. The bone edges are then smoothed with a suitable burr or file.

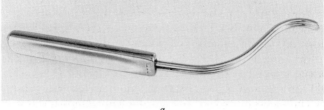

a

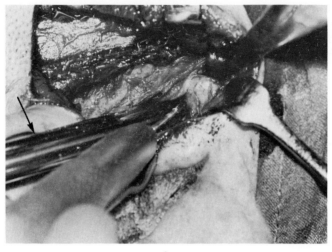

b

Fig. 7.7. a, Temporomandibular joint retractor (Caterham Surgical Supplies Ltd, Surrey). *b,* The temporomandibular joint retractor (arrowed) in position, protecting the soft tissues and acting as a guide to excising the articular surface of the condyle.

5. The meniscus now is free from the lateral aspect of the condyle and capsule. The posterior attachment is clamped with a suitable pair of fine forceps, as close to the edge of the meniscus as possible and drawn backwards. It now should lie over the recontoured condyle. It is maintained in this relationship by the excision of a wedge of tissue from the posterior attachment and suture of the cut edges together. The lateral border of the meniscus is sutured to remaining lateral condylar attachment and periosteum. The position of the meniscus in function now may be checked manually by opening and closing the jaw.

6. The capsule is repaired and the operative site closed in layers. No dressing need be applied but some surgeons prefer to use a pressure-pad bandage for 24 hours. The pledget is extracted from the external auditory meatus and the ear inspected for blood clot. If this is not removed, it may be responsible for considerable postoperative discomfort.

The patient is advised to rest the jaw and keep to a very soft diet over the succeeding two weeks. Then, gradually, normal function may be resumed. Exercises, such as those described on p. 84 may be helpful. The occlusion frequently is altered in the immediate postoperative period but the temptation to treat it by grinding the teeth should be resisted as generally it corrects itself.

Condylotomy

A condylotomy is a procedure in which the neck of the condyle is surgically fractured, usually allowing some forward and medial displacement of the condylar fragment. The rationale behind the treatment is that it allows the condyle to assume a new functional position in relation to the displaced meniscus.

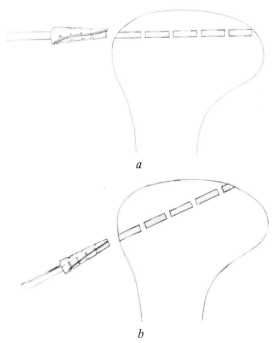

a

b

Fig. 7.8. Excision of the condylar surface. *a*, Correct; *b*, Incorrect.

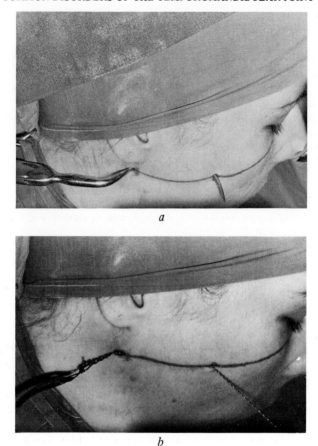

Fig. 7.9. Closed condylotomy. *a,* The Kostecka awl passing deep to the neck of the condyle, through the sigmoid notch to emerge anteriorly. *b,* The Kostecka has been withdrawn, pulling with it a Gigli saw.

The procedure may be carried out by either an open or a closed technique, and it was the latter that was first developed by Ward (1961) as a modification of the closed ramus section (Kostecka, 1928).

Closed Condylotomy
Under a general anaesthetic, the mouth is opened as widely as possible bringing the head of the condyle up to the crest of the eminentia articularis. A reference line is drawn from a point a finger's breadth below the ear lobe to the infra-orbital margin (*Fig.* 7.9*a*). A stab incision

is made through the skin at the posterior point and a Kostecka awl passed deep to the neck of the condyle into the sigmoid notch. The pointed end of the instrument is kept in contact with the bone, to emerge through a second stab incision over the reference line. A Gigli saw is pulled back with the awl (*Fig. 7.9b*) and the condylar neck divided. To prevent too great a displacement of the condylar fragment, the attempt is made to leave the medial and lateral periosteum intact. However, reporting an investigation into the technique on three cadavar specimens, Buckerfield (1978) concluded that it might be difficult to introduce the Kostecka awl subperiostially on the medial side, and that the final sawing movement and the removal of the Gigli saw may divide the lateral periosteum.

No postoperative immobilization of the jaws is necessary unless there is severe discomfort or disruption of the occlusion, but it is frequently necessary to carry out minor cuspal adjustments of the teeth within a month of the operation.

A criticism of the technique is that it is a 'blind' procedure. There is the possibility that the external carotid artery might be damaged and, indeed, in a series of 141 cases reported by Banks and Mackenzie (1975), there were 9 cases of excessive haematoma in the region of the posterior border of the mandibular ramus and one operation had to be abandoned because of haemorrhage. However, since it is a closed procedure, haemostasis was eventually obtained in each case by means of hot packs and external pressure. Damage to the maxillary artery is again a possibility and here there is the potential danger of haematoma compressing the pharynx and occluding the airway.

Laceration of the facial nerve will cause persistent facial weakness and it occurred in 6 cases of a series of 250 reported by Tasanen and Lamberg (1974). This complication was not noted by Banks and Mackenzie, but paraesthesia of the inferior dental nerve was a problem in 15 cases.

In spite of these potential hazards, closed condylotomy has met with undoubted success in many cases of pain and dysfunction of the temporomandibular joint which have failed to respond to conservative therapy. In Banks and Mackenzie's series, approximately 45 per cent were cured and the same number improved. Only 9·5 per cent of the patients were evaluated as no better or worse. Other series (Campbell, 1965; Sada, 1967) have produced comparable results.

Open Condylotomy

Division of the neck of the condyle may be carried out via the preauricular incision described earlier. While protecting the soft tissues with a temporomandibular joint retractor, a complete transverse section of the bone below the capsule is made. The cut, which is the width of the burr (2–3 mm), is usually seen to collapse and completely close, the parallel bony surfaces lying together. If the burr cut is made as high as possible adjacent to the capsule, then some part of the lateral pterygoid muscle will remain attached to the condylar fragment and some to the upper part of the neck of the condyle. This avoids unwanted displacement of the articular fragment.

Perhaps the most important advantage of the open procedure, however, is the opportunity it gives to inspect the joint. This allows a change or modification of the operation according to the findings. Thus, a high condylectomy may be performed, or the surgeon might elect to be conservative and simply reposition the displaced meniscus.

CHAPTER 8

CONCLUSION

The views expressed in this book have been based on the hypothesis that the common disorders of the temporomandibular joint are due to trauma. This may be through an acute traumatic incident, stress-induced neuromuscular overload or both.

Consequently, the term 'mandibular stress syndrome' has been proposed. Treatment, it has been argued, should be aimed at reducing or eliminating the overload.

By careful analysis and planning along the lines described in the preceeding chapters, the majority of cases may be managed with a high degree of success; but there will be disappointments and failures. These may be due to poor patient compliance with the treatment advocated, misdiagnosis or faulty clinical technique. However, the objective of this approach is to provide a rational explanation for the clinical findings which should account for the apparent diversity of the many widely practised treatments.

The preparation for the text of this book required a thorough search of the vast literature pertaining to the temporomandibular joint. It emerged, that in the past, many of the difficulties in the understanding of the problem have been due to an inadequate appreciation of the anatomy of the joint, especially its meniscus. With the advent of the new imaging techniques this has largely been overcome. The meniscus should be regarded not as a disc but as a movable, flexible diaphragm, dividing the articulation into two compartments. Thus, it serves not only as a protective cushion between the articular surfaces absorbing much of the functional load, but also renders the joint exceptionally versatile. It facilitates the complex rotational and sliding motions of the condyle during normal jaw function.

When the normal relationship of the meniscus to the bony articulating surfaces becomes disturbed then a dysfunction occurs. If this is unresolved, then, eventually, further more damaging changes may follow.

There are two important factors in the management of temporomandibular joint disorders that are worth stressing yet again. The first is that the patient must be given an explanation of the problem. Only when this is readily understood does the prognosis become favourable and getting the message across is dependent upon the second factor, time.

The assessment of a disorder and especially the psychic aspects of its treatment may require many prolonged consultations. Progress may be slow and perseverence is essential to explain the problem to the patient over and over again. There are no quick and simple remedies. The clinician must therefore be able and prepared to devote the facilities and time commensurate with the kind of logical approach that has been recommended. In this way the management of mandibular stress syndrome is not merely a chore but a rewarding experience for both patient and doctor.

REFERENCES

Agerberg G. (1974) Maximal mandibular movements in young men and women. *Swed. Dent. J.* **67**, 81.

Agerberg G. and Lundberg M. (1971) Changes in the temporomandibular joint after surgical treatment. A radiologic follow-up study. *Oral Surg.* **32**, 865.

Anderson Q. N. and Katzberg R. W. (1094) Loose bodies of the temporomandibular joint: arthrographic diagnosis. *Skeletal Radiol.* **11**, 42.

Annadale T. (1887) Displacement of the inter-articular cartilage of the lower jaw and its treatment by operation. *Lancet* **1**, 411.

Banks P. and Mackenzie I. (1975) Condylotomy. A clinical and experimental appraisal of a surgical technique. *J. Maxillofac. Surg.* **3** (3), 170.

Barbenel J. C. (1974) The mechanics of the temporomandibular joint; a theoretical and electromyographical study. *J. Oral Rehabil.* **1**, 19.

Bean L. R., Omnell K. A. and Oberg T. (1977) Comparisons between radiologic observations and macroscopic tissue change in temporomandibular joints. *Dento-maxillofac. Radiol.* **6**, 90.

Beemsterboer P. L., McNamara D. C., Holden S. et al. (1976) The effect of the bite plane splint on the electromyographic silent period duration. *J. Oral Rehabil.* **3**, 349.

Berry D. C. (1960) The relationship between some anatomical features of the human mandibular condyle and its appearance on radiographs. *Arch. Oral Biol.* **2**, 203.

Berry D. C. and Watkinson A. C. (1978) Mandibular dysfunction and incisor relationship. *Br. Dent. J.* **144**, 74–77.

Berry D. C. and Yemm R. (1974) A further study of facial skin temperature in patients with mandibular dysfunction. *J. Oral Rehabil.* **1**, 255.

Bessette R., Bishop B. and Mohl N. (1971) Duration of masseteric silent period in patients with temporomandibular joint syndrome. *J. Appl. Psychol.* **30**, 864.

Blackman S. (1963) Radiography of the temporomandibular joint. *Br. J. Oral Surg.* **1**, 132.

Blackwood H. J. J. (1962) Disease of the mandibular joint in the child; Oral pathology in the child. *NY Int. Acad. Oral Pathol.* p. 64.

Blackwood H. J. J. (1963) Arthritis of the mandibular joint. *Br. Dent. J.* **115**, 317.

Blackwood H. J. J. (1966a) Cellular remodelling in articular tissue. *J. Dent. Res.* **45**, 400.

Blackwood H. J. J. (1966b) Study of the growth of the mandibular condyle of the rat. Studies with tritiated thymidine. *Arch. Oral Biol.* **11**, 493.

Blackwood H. J. J. (1976) The mandibular joint; development, structure and function. In: Cohen B. and Kramer I. A. H. (ed.), *Scientific Foundations of Dentistry.* London, Heinemann, p. 592.

Bloch F., Hansen W. W. and Packard (1946) Nuclear induction. *Physiol. Rev.* **69**, 127.

Boering C. (1966) Arthrosis deformans van het kaakgewricht. Diss. Groningen, Drukkerij Van Dendern.

Buckerfield J. P. (1978) The applied anatomy of closed condylotomy. *Br. J. Oral Surg.* **15**, 245.

Campbell W. (1965) Clinical and radiographical investigations of the mandibular joints. *Br. J. Radiol.* **28**, 401.

Coin C. G. (1974) Tomography of the temporomandibular joint. *Med. Radiogr. Photogr.* **50**, 26.

Costen J. B. (1934) A syndrome of ear and sinus symptoms dependent upon disturbed functions of the temporomandibular joint. *Ann. Otol. Rhinol. Laryngol.* **43**, I.

Dingmann R. O. and Grabb W. C. (1966) Intra-capsular temporomandibular joint arthroplasty. *Plast. Reconstr. Surg.* **38**, 179.

Editorial (1977) *Br. Med. J.* **2**, 979.

Editorial (1973) *Lancet* **2**, 1131.

Farrar W. B. (1978) Characteristics of the condylar path in internal derangements of the temporomandibular joint. *J. Prosthet. Dent.* **39**, 319.

Farrar W. B. and McCarty W. L. (1979) Inferior joint space arthrography and characteristics of condylar paths in internal derangements of the TMJ. *J. Prosthet. Dent.* **41**, 548.

Freeman M. A. R. and Kempson G. E. (1973) In: Freeman M. A. R. (ed.), *Load Carriage. Adult Articular Cartilage.* London, Pitman Medical, pp. 228–246.

Gibson T., Burry H. C., Poswillo D. et al. (1976) Effect of intra-articular corticosteroid injections on primate cartilage. *Ann. Rheum. Dis.* **36**, 74.

Goharian R. K. and Neff C. A. (1980) Effect of occlusal retainers on temporomandibular joint and facial pain. *J. Prosthet. Dent.* **44**, 206.

Goodman P., Greene C. S. and Laskin D. M. (1976) Response of patients with myofascial pain-dysfunction syndrome to mock equilibration. *J. Am. Dent. Assoc.* **92**, 755.

Greene C. S. (1973) A survey of current professional concepts and opinions about M.P.D. syndrome. *J. Am. Dent. Assoc.* **86**, 128.

Greene C. S. and Laskin D. M. (1972) Splint therapy for myofascial pain dysfunction syndrome: a comparative study. *J. Am. Dent. Assoc.* **84**, 624.

Guralnick W., Kaban L. B. and Merril R. G. (1978) Temporomandibular joint afflictions. *N. Engl. J. Med.* **299**, 123.

Hamerman D., Rosenburg L. C. and Schubert M. (1970) Diarthrodial joints revised. *J. Bone Joint Surg.* **62**, 725.

Harris M. (1985) Medical or physical management of facial muscle and joint pain. *Br. Dent. J.* **158**, 227.

Helkimo M. (1976) Epidemiological surveys of dysfunction of the masticatory system. *Oral Sci. Rev.* **7**, 54.

Helms C. A., Morrish R. B., Kircos L. T. et al. (1982) Computed tomography of the meniscus of the temporomandibular joint: preliminary observations. *Radiology* **145**, 719.

REFERENCES

Helms C. A., Richardson M. L., Moon K. L. et al. (1984) Nuclear magnetic resonance imaging of the temporomandibular joint: preliminary observations. *J. Craniomand. Pract.* 2, 219.

Henny F. A. (1969) Surgical treatment of painful temporomandibular joint. *J. Am. Dent. Assoc.* 79, 171.

Henny F. A. and Baldridge O. L. (1957) Condylectomy for persistently painful temporomandibular joint. *J. Oral Surg.* 15, 24.

Hollander J. L., Brown E. M. jun., Jesser R. A. et al. (1951) Hydrocortisone and cortisone injected into arthritic joints. *J. Am. Dent. Assoc.* 147, 1629.

Horton C. P. (1953) The treatment of arthritic temporomandibular joints by intra-articular injection of hydrocortisone. *Oral Surg.* 6, 826.

Juniper R. P. (1981) The superior pterygoid muscle? *Br. J. Oral Surg.* 19, 121.

Juniper R. P. (1984) Temporomandibular joint dysfunction: A theory based upon electromyographic studies of the lateral pterygoid muscle. *Br. J. Oral Maxillofac. Surg.* 22, 1.

Katzberg R. W., Dolwick M. F., Helms C. A. et al. (1980) Arthrotomography of the temporomandibular joint. *Am. J. Roentgenol.* 134, 995.

Katzberg R. W., Keith D. A., Guralnick W. C. et al. (1982) Correlation of condylar mobility and arthrotomography in patients with internal derangements of the temporomandibular joint. *Oral Surg.* 54, 622.

Katzberg R. W., Keith D. A., Guralnick W. C. et al. (1983a) Internal derangements and arthritis of the temporomandibular joint. *Radiology* 146, 107.

Katzberg R. W., Keith D. A., Ten Eick W. R. et al. (1983b) Internal derangements of the temporomandibular joint: an assessment of condylar position in centric occlusion. *J. Prosthet. Dent.* 49, 250.

Katzberg R. W., Schenck J., Roberts D. et al. (1985) Magnetic resonance imaging of the TMJ and meniscus. *Oral Surg.* 59(4); 332.

Kostecka F. (1928) Surgical correction of protrusion of the lower and upper jaws. *J. Am. Dent. Assoc.* 15, 362.

Laskin D. M. (1969) Etiology of the pain dysfunction syndrome. *J. Am. Dent. Assoc.* 79, 147.

Lauterber P. (1973) Image formation by induced local interactions: examples employing nuclear magnetic resonance. *Nature* 242, 190.

Littleton J. T. (1976) *Tomography: Physical Principles and Clinical Application.* Baltimore: Williams & Wilkins.

Macalister A. D. (1954) A microscopic survey of the human temporomandibular joint. *NZ Dent. J.* 50, 161.

MacMahon B. and Pugh T. F. (1970) *Epidemiology. Principles and Methods.* Boston, Little, Brown.

McQueen W. W. (1937) Radiography of the temporomandibular articulation. *Minneapolis District Dent. J.* 21, 28.

Manzione J. V., Seltzer S. E., Katzberg R. W. et al. (1982) Direct sagittal computed tomography of the temporomandibular joint. *Am. J. Nuclear Roentgenol.* 3, 677.

Manzione J. V., Seltzer S. E., Katzberg R. W. et al. (1983) Direct sagittal computed tomography of the temporomandibular joint. *Am. J. Roentgenol.* **140**, 165.

Manzione J. V., Katzberg R. W., Brodsky G. L. et al. (1984a) Internal derangements of the temporomandibular joint: diagnosis by direct sagittal computed tomography. *Radiology* **150**, 111.

Manzione J. V., Katzberg R. W. and Manzione T. J. (1984b) Internal derangements of the temporomandibular joint: I. Normal anatomy, physiology and pathophysiology. *Int. J. Periodontal. Rest. Dent.* **4**, 9.

Manzione J. V., Tallents R., Katzberg R. W. et al. (1984c) Arthrographically guided splint therapy for recapturing the temporomandibular joint meniscus. *Oral Surg.* **57**, 235.

Manzione J. V., Katzberg R. W. and Manzione T. J. (1984d) Internal derangements of the temporomandibular joint: II. Diagnosis by arthrography and computed tomography. *Int. J. Periodontal. Rest. Dent.* **4**, 17.

Matthews M. P. and Moffett B. C. jun. (1974) Histologic maturation and initial ageing of the human temporomandibular joint. *J. Dent. Res.* **53**, 246.

Mayne J. G. and Hatch G. S. (1969) Arthritis of the temporomandibular joint. *J. Am. Dent. Assoc.* **79**, 125.

Miles A. E. W. and Dawson J. A. (1962) Elastic fibres in the articular fibrous tissue of some joints. *Arch. Oral Biol.* **7**, 249.

Moss A. L. and Rankow R. (1968) The role of the functional matrix in mandibular growth. *Angle Orthod.* **38**, 95.

Muir H. (1977) Molecular approach to the understanding of osteoarthrosis. *Ann. Rheum. Dis.* **36**, 199.

Muir H., Maroudas A. and Wingham J. (1969) The correlation of fixed negative charge with glycosaminoglycan content of human articular cartilage. *Biochim. Biophys. Acta* **177**, 494.

Nevakari K. (1960) 'Elapsio Praecenticularis' of the temporomandibular joint. A pantomographic study of the so-called physiological subluxation. *Acta Odontol. Scand.* **18**, 123.

Nörgaard F. (1947) Temporomandibular arthrography. Thesis. Copenhagen, Munksgaard.

Oberg T., Carlson G. E. and Fajers M. (1971) The temporomandibular joint. A morphogenic study on human autopsy material. *Acta Odontol. Scand.* **29**, 439.

Ogus H. D. (1975) Rheumatoid arthritis of the temporomandibular joint. *Br. J. Oral Surg.* **12**, 275.

Ogus H. D. (1978) Degenerative disease of the temporomandibular joint and pain-dysfunction syndrome. *J. R. Soc. Med.* **71**, 748.

Ogus H. D. (1979) Degenerative disease of the temporomandibular joint in young persons. *Br. J. Oral Surg.* **17**, 17.

Poswillo D. E. (1970) Experimental investigation of the effects of intra-articular hydrocortisone and high condylectomy on the mandibular condyle. *Oral Surg.* **30**, 161.

REFERENCES

Purcell E. M., Torrey H. C. and Pound R. V. (1946) Resonance absorption by nuclear magnetic moments in a solid. *Physiol. Rev.* **69**, 37.

Radin E. L., Paul I. L. and Rose R. M. (1972) Role of mechanical factors in the pathogenesis of primary osteoarthrosis. *Lancet* **1**, 519.

Ralph J. P. (1977) Stress distribution in the mandibular condyle under simulated occlusal loads. *Int. Assoc. Dent. Res.* Abstracts No. 190.

Ramfjord S. P. and Ash M. jun. (1971) *Occlusion.* Philadelphia, Saunders, p. 11.

Rees L. A. (1954) The structure and function of the mandibular joint. *Br. Dent. J.* **96**, 125.

Ricketts R. M. (1975) Mechanisms of mandibular growth; a series of enquiries on the growth of the mandible. In: McNamara J. A. (ed.), *Determinants of Mandibular Form and Growth.* Monogr. 4, Ann Arbor Centre for Human Growth and Development p. 77.

Rothwell P. S. (1972) Personality and temporomandibular joint dysfunction. *Oral Surg.* **34**, 734.

Rugh J. D. and Solberg W. K. (1976) Psychological implications in temporomandibular pain and dysfunction. *Oral Sci. Rev.* **7**, 3.

Sada V. (1967) Experience in surgical treatment of temporomandibular joint arthrosis by the Ward technique. *Trans. Congress of the First Int. Assoc. Oral Surgeons,* 265.

Salter R. B., Gross A. and Hall J. H. (1967) Hydrocortisone arthropathy. An experimental investigation. *Can. Med. Assoc. J.* **97**, 374.

Sartoris D. J., Neumann C. H. and Riley R. W. (1984) The temporomandibular joint: true sagittal computed tomography with meniscus visualization. *Radiology* **150**, 250.

Schwartz L. (1956) A temporomandibular joint pain-dysfunction syndrome. *J. Chron. Dis.* **3**, 284.

Schwartz H. C. and Kendrick R. W. (1984) Internal derangements of the temporomandibular joint: Description of clinical syndromes. *Oral Surg.* **58**, 24.

Smith N. J. D. and Harris M. (1970) Radiology of the temporomandibular joint and condylar head. *Br. Dent. J.* 361.

Sperber G. M. (1976) *Craniofacial Embryology.* 2nd ed. Bristol, Wright.

Standlee J. P., Caputo A. A. and Ralph J. P. (1977) Stress trajectories within the mandible under occlusal loads. *J. Dent. Res.* **56**, 1297.

Standlee J. P., Caputo A. A. and Ralph J. P. (1979) Stress transfer to the mandible during anterior guidance and group function eccentric movements. *J. Prosthet. Dent.* **41**, 35.

Standlee J. P., Caputo A. A. and Ralph J. P. (1981) The condyle as a stress distributing component of the temporomandibular joint. *J. Oral Rehabil.* **9**, 23.

Stanson A. W. and Baker H. L. (1976) Routine tomography of the temporomandibular joint. *Radiol. Clin. N.Am.* **14**, 105.

Tasanen A. and Lamberg M. A. (1974) Closed condylotomy in the treatment of osteoarthrosis of the temporomandibular joint. *Int. J. Oral Surg.* **3**, 102.

Thomson H. (1971) Mandibular dysfunction syndrome. *Br. Dent. J.* **130**, 187.

Thompson J. R., Christiansen E., Hasso A. N. et al. (1984) Temporo-mandibular joints: high resolution computed tomographic evaluation. *Radiology* **150**, 105.

Toller P. A. (1969) Transpharyngeal radiography for arthritis of the mandibular condyle. *Br. J. Oral Surg.* **7**, 47.

Toller P. A. (1973) Osteoarthrosis of the mandibular condyle. *Br. Dent. J.* **134**, 223.

Toller P. A. (1974a) Temporomandibular capsular rearrangement. *Br. J. Oral Surg.* **11**, 207.

Toller P. A. (1974b) Temporomandibular arthropathy. *Proc. R. Soc. Med.* **67**, 153.

Toller P. A. (1974c) Opaque arthrography of the temporomandibular joint. *Int. J. Oral Surg.* **3**, 17.

Toller P. A. (1976) Non-surgical treatment of dysfunctions of the temporomandibular joint. *Oral Sci. Rev.* **7**, 70.

Toller P. A. (1977a) Ultrastructure of the condylar articular surface in severe mandibular pain-dysfunction syndrome. *Int. J. Oral Surg.* **6**, 279.

Toller P. A. (1977b) Use and misuse of intra-articular corticosteroids in the treatment of temporomandibular joint pain. *Proc. R. Soc. Med.* **70**, 461.

Toller P. A. and Wilcox J. H. (1978) Ultrastructure of the articular surface of the condyle in temporomandibular arthropathy. *Oral Surg.* **45**, 232.

Updegrave W. J. (1968) In: Schwartz L. and Chayes C. M. (ed.), *Facial Pain and Mandibular Dysfunction*. Philadelphia, Saunders.

Ward T. G. (1961) Surgery of the mandibular joint. *Ann. R. Coll. Surg. Engl.* **28**, 139.

Weightman B. O., Freeman M. A. R. and Swanson S. A. V. (1973) Fatigue of articular cartilage. *Nature* **224**, 303.

Weinberg L. A. (1972) Correlation of temporomandibular joint dysfunction with radiographic findings. *J. Prosthet. Dent.* **28**, 519.

Weinberg L. A. (1977) Evaluation of stress in temporomandibular joint pain-dysfunction syndrome. *J. Prosthet. Dent.* **38**, 192.

Weinberg L. A. (1979) Role in condylar position in TMJ dysfunction-pain syndrome. *J. Prosthet. Dent.* **41**, 636.

Wilkes C. (1978) Arthrography of temporomandibular joint in patients with TMJ pain dysfunction syndrome. *Minn. Med.* **61**, 645.

Wyke B. D. (1976) Temporomandibular articular pain. In: Cohen B. and Kramer I. A. H. (ed.), *Scientific Foundations of Dentistry*. London, Heinemann, p. 293.

Yemm R. (1976) Neurophysiologic studies of temporomandibular joint dysfunction. *Oral Sci. Rev.* **7**, 31.

Zarb G. A. and Thompson G. W. (1975) The treatment of patients with temporomandibular joint pain-dysfunction syndrome. *J. Canad. Dent. Assoc.* **7**, 410.

INDEX